A Journey
To Vibrant Health

by Dr. Rachel Northern
Family Wellness Doctor

Brian & Angela,
May Vibrant
Health always
be yours!
Dr. Rachel

Northern Light Care
Johnsburg, Illinois

A Journey to Vibrant Health

Published by Northern Light Care
2302 Johnsburg Road #1
Johnsburg, Illinois 60051 USA

Printed in the United States of America

ISBN-13: 978-0692808375
ISBN-10: 069280837X

Cover design by Jake Gallegos, New Freedom Design

Library of Congress Control Number: 2016920338

DISCLAIMER AND/OR LEGAL NOTICES
   This book is for information and educational purposes only. The information contained herein does not constitute or replace the chiropractic or healthcare advice of a chiropractic physicians or other medical professional. This book is not intended to assist with self-diagnosis or treatment; therefore, any decisions regarding your healthcare should be made in consultation with your chiropractic physician or other medical professional. Nothing in this book is a guarantee of outcome. While the author took pains to present accurate and up-to date information, neither Dr. Rachel Northern, D.C., or Northern Light Care, Inc. is responsible for errors or omissions.
   While the publisher and author have used their best efforts in preparing this book, they make no representations or warranties with respect to the accuracy or completeness of the contents of this book. Neither the publisher nor the author shall be liable for any loss of profit or any other commercial damages, including but not limited to special, incidental, consequential, or other damages. The purchaser or reader of this publication assumes responsibility for the use of these materials and information. Adherence to all applicable laws and regulations, both advertising and all other aspects of doing business in the United States or any other jurisdiction, is the sole responsibility of the purchaser or reader.

www.TheDoctorInYou.com

Contents

Foreword by Dr. Rob Jackson.. iii

One   A Healthy, Vibrant You Awaits......................... 1

Two   Your Body: OWNERS ~ Investments That Pay Off....... 12

Three   Oxygen: You Are What You Breathe........................... 22

Four   Want Vitality? Water *Works!* 26

Five   Nutrients: Some Unexpected Insights........................... 32

Six   Nutrients That Heal Your Body......................... 47

Seven   Exercise Your Passion! 63

Eight   Rest to Renew You 68

Nine   Social Health Externally That Rejuvenates You
Internally 74

Ten   Spiritual Health: Meditate on This and Be Uplifted .. 101

About the Author **107**

Foreword
by Dr. Rob Jackson

In her new book *A Journey to Vibrant Health*, Dr. Rachel Northern does a tremendous job of taking an in-depth look at our cultural beliefs on how we define health and healthcare.

Just like many of her readers and patients, Dr. Rachel has had a history of personal health care issues that she had to address while going through her childhood, becoming a wife and mother, and then becoming a practicing doctor.

These presenting symptoms or issues stem from the habits, cultures, and beliefs that so many of us grew up with. But we have found that they do not serve our needs or wants today. Due to social media and the availability of alternative information on the Web, people are questioning the outdated western style of allopathic (MD) medicine.

In the pages ahead, Dr. Rachel shares healing insights on everything from eating and the habits we have created over the past fifty years, to the choices we can make regarding drinking water, types of lip balm, insecticides, and everything in between. All of these can have either a positive or negative impact on our own and our family's health. And Dr. Rachel reveals exactly what and why.

In each chapter she takes on an important health care issue, and then provides detailed information with a step-by-step solution for those who want to tackle that specific subject.

She also shares up-to-date and personal health care choices that can help those who have issues or concerns and are looking for answers.

I recommend *A Journey to Vibrant Health* as an important read for anyone who wants direct and simple answers to the health care questions that so many of us have today, answers that can be implemented right away without being sold anything in the process.

The information she provides is simple, yet detailed and refreshing from beginning to end.

—Dr. Rob Jackson
President,
Back Talk Systems, Inc.
231 Violet Street, Unit 140
Golden, Colorado 80401
www.BackTalkSystems.com

ℛ   One

A Healthy, Vibrant You Awaits

According to DNA, you should live about 120 years.

Surprised? Fact is, you are *designed* to be healthy. You are designed to heal from illness.

For example, think about your fingerprints. Everybody has his or her own. They're all individual. Unique. Now, if your finger gets a papercut, it takes around seven days for that papercut to heal completely. And when it heals, the body knows how to put those ridges right where they're supposed to be. It's amazing. Your fingerprint grows back exactly the same as it was before the papercut.

Your body does the same internally. It knows how to heal your organs and the rest of what makes you up.

It knows how to make itself healthy. We are self-healing, self-regulating, adaptable beings.

What *IS* Health?

I ask every new chiropractic patient who comes through my door, "What is health?"

Most of them are stumped. They've never really thought about it.

That's part of why our culture of health is what it is: We are what we think about. If we don't think about what health is, and evaluate it, we aren't going to truly know.

After a pause, patients generally answer, "I guess health is feeling good. Being able to do what I want to do."

Feeling good is not enough of an answer. Here's why.

Recently my friend was feeling fine. Then her eye color changed to yellow. The next thing you know, she was diagnosed with pancreatic cancer.

It's a similar situation with the onset of diabetes. You feel fine, and then all of a sudden you're peeing a lot, or craving sweets. Next thing you know you've been diagnosed with diabetes.

The sensation of feeling things physically is only about 10 to 15 percent of the nervous system. If we rely only on that small percentage of sensory input to tell us how we're doing, that's not a good basis for deciding we're healthy.

Don't get me wrong—healthy people feel good. But unhealthy people can feel good too.

So we can't rely on how we "feel." It's just not a good standard.

Instead, what I talk to patients about is **function**. Most patients who initially come to me are in discomfort or pain. After a number of chiropractic sessions, we do re-evaluations. At that point they might be "feeling" good again, but I'll still see that they can't rotate their body parts within a normal range or they have skin or digestion issues.

Does your body function well? Does it function the way it's designed to?

The New "Normal"

I examine patients and ask, "Do you get headaches?"

They commonly reply, "I just get normal headaches."

Then I have to educate them. I say, "Actually, the body shouldn't have headaches. What if I told you that headaches are not normal?"

"Oh" commonly follows.

Normal doesn't mean healthy.

I often ask, "Are you having regular bowel movements?"

Many patients reply, "I go every two or three days. That's how I've always been. It's normal."

I respond, "No. That's not normal. It means something isn't functioning right. It means something isn't healthy."

Much of our society today is overweight. And since so many are overweight, that makes us feel like it's okay. That's the norm.

Millions of people now have illnesses and diseases. Nobody has just one thing wrong with them anymore. You don't just have asthma; you also have two or three other health issues. But because the changes to our health have been gradual, we've acclimated to living in ill health. Since it's a slow progression, we don't see how deadly it is.

We're frogs in a huge pot that has started to boil.

You know that story of the frog and the pot of water. You put a frog in a pot of cool water, then slowly increase the heat under the pot. The frog gradually acclimates to the change. Eventually the frog dies because it gets boiled to death.

That's our society. We're in that pot of water. We are at crisis.

We rank around thirty-third on healthy nation evaluations. There are thirty-two nations healthier than us! Yet, we spend the most amount of money on health.

We can no longer accept society-normal. We have to find our way back to healthy-normal.

Healthy-normal is no headaches. Healthy-normal is a good balance of muscle tone and good rotation. Healthy-normal is regular, daily bowel movements and other bodily functions.

But health is even more than that. Health affects every aspect of our lives. If our physical body is not working right, it affects our mental state, which in return affects our relationships.

For example, if you have a headache, you're less focused to handle your job duties. Or when you get home and your kids are playing around, you don't have the patience that you normally would have without the headache.

If you just had a death in the family or a relationship breakup, you might wake in the morning with a lack of energy and possibly with physical pain.

The mind, body, and heart are inseparably interconnected.

Health, then, is not merely "feeling good" or the absence of disease. It is much more. **Health is vibrant physical, mental, social, and spiritual functioning and well-being.**

With that definition in mind, health is something we have to focus on and work for.

The Role of Culture

In today's world, we're constantly told what to think and what to do. In fact, we're relentlessly bombarded by advertising—online, on television, radio, in the grocery store, drugstore, at movie theaters, in restaurants, in taxi cabs. We're conditioned to go with the flow. Go with the culture. This is normal.

That's led us to our national health crisis today.

We've come to see our food and lifestyle as, "It is what it is." Relatively few people actually take time to consider it. They're not consciously thinking, "Is this even right?"

They get up every morning, stressed out, and they believe, "This is how I have to do it. Everybody else is stressed out with their finances. Everybody else is stressed out about their jobs. They're all stressed about their health. Every one of them is running their kids around like crazy to sports practices and games."

We're surrounded with the same kind of thinking, and we'll continue to think that way, unless somebody steps up and challenges us on our way of thinking. **Or** unless we have a health crisis. **Or** a family crisis, such as a child gets addicted to drugs.

Unfortunately, many times it's when the big "ah-ha" pain moment comes does someone think, "Maybe we should reassess this."

So we have to stop, look at our culture, and think, "Okay, just because it's happening to someone else, does it have to happen to me? Does this have to be my journey too?"

We need to take responsibility for what information we let in as fact. When we do, we can have amazing epiphanies, and we can see the contradictions. We can see how hectic and chaotic and unhealthy our culture has become.

We can realize, "This isn't right, and I shouldn't be doing it. This isn't healthy for me."

The Role of Modern Medicine

As a nation we spend the most money on pharmaceuticals. We consume 80 percent of the pharmaceuticals that are produced on the planet. We're surrounded by non-foods and other toxins. And we just take it in.

When symptoms arise, we go to a medical doctor for a pill.

Don't get me wrong. I don't put down MDs at all. We need MDs. If I get into a car accident, they are fabulous at crisis care. If I have appendicitis or any emergency that needs immediate attention, they are phenomenal at doing that. That's what they are trained for, and that's what the drugs can do. They can get the body to survive.

However, when it comes to preventative care and long-term maintenance of the body, that's where MDs' schooling and tools may not be the best option. Healthy people don't go to the doctor. So most MDs don't know how to maintain healthy people, and they don't see the benefits of healthy lifestyles. All they see are people who are in crisis or sick.

Most MDs don't think like us holistic doctors. In contrast, Holistic doctors provide preventative care and long-term maintenance. We see people who are healthy and trying to maintain their health.

One of my teachers/mentors told a story to an audience to describe MD work versus what we do. He said, "MDs are like firefighters. Your house is on fire, you want to save the house, and they'll do whatever they need to do. They'll break a window. They'll cave in the door. They'll douse the fire and save the house, and save whoever is in the house. They'll try to save whatever they can. But afterward, they don't know what to do! Afterward, the firefighters leave. That's when the maintenance people come in, and they clean it up.

"We holistic practitioners are like the maintenance people. We're like carpenters who come in and make sure we keep the house functioning long-term. That's what we holistic people do. We want to maintain the house."

If somebody calls me and thinks they're having a heart attack, I'm going to send them to the ER. I'm not trained to help that. I know my place in the system. I respect that. Each group of doctors, MD and holistic, has its own purpose.

Now, I've come across some MDs who've realized that their world is upside down. They recognize, "Wow, this is wrong!" And they've seen the power of teaching people how to eat properly and avoid stress, the way nature intended. They've fully realized that our bodies are amazing, and that we need to trust our bodies to heal themselves.

Those few have become aware of their role in culture.

I always say, "I don't heal anything. I don't cure anything. The body is amazingly built." We've lost faith in our bodies, in the way that we're made. Allopathic (modern medicine) is all about treating the symptom, or "What can we do to patch it?" We holistic practitioners are saying, "No. The body is wise. The body is trying to communicate something. We need to find out what's going on and try to restore that balance, restore that communication, restore whatever is in need of restoring, so that the *body* can heal that area, recalibrate, or do whatever it needs to do."

Due to culture, we've lost faith in our bodies. We need to get back that faith. And we must take the blinders off our culture. We must crawl out of the boiling pot.

Our human bodies have been healing themselves for millennia—long before the rise of modern medicine.

"Imagine My Surprise"

By now you've guessed that I have quite a passion for helping people to be healthy.

Everybody thinks because I'm a so-called health guru today, "Oh, it's easy for her." But, I didn't grow up this way. How I arrived here is actually a little surprising, even to me. My own illness finally opened my eyes.

Here's what happened.

As I grew up, I didn't eat a lot of fruits and vegetables. There were usually a few shriveled up oranges and apples in the bottom of the refrigerator, and I remember broccoli being smothered in cheese. My parents weren't really into eating healthy. There were just so busy, they didn't have time.

My freshman year of high school, my breakfast was Hershey's chocolate milk—every morning. I can't believe I made it through! (Though no wonder I had anxiety throughout sophomore year!)

When I was twelve, I had episodes of sharp ear pain that kept coming and going. My mom took me to a medical doctor who couldn't see anything wrong—no ear infection, no problems. One finally gave us ear drops and sent us on our way. The episodes continued to come and go.

Then my dad took me to an urgent care center. They did blood work but didn't see anything wrong. So they dismissed what I was saying and asked my dad if I was faking it or needed attention. That was completely not me because I was an only child, got plenty of attention, *and* I hated missing school—I was one of those studious kids.

Listening to them tell my dad I could be faking the sharp pain, I realized, "Wow, these doctors who are supposed to know everything *don't* know everything! I have an issue, and they don't have answers!"

Finally my mom brought me to one more medical doctor. Like the others, he said, "I don't see anything wrong."

My disillusion about allopathic medicine (MD medicine—treat all symptoms pharmacologically) was a turning point.

Even at the age of twelve, I advocated for myself and my health. I told him, "Listen, this is not fake. This is real. I *am* experiencing this. You're just not finding anything."

He said, "Okay, you're right. I did notice some tension in your neck. Let's try a chiropractor."

When the chiropractor evaluated me, we found that half the vertebras in my neck were not in the right place. Instead of getting a headache or neck pain, I was getting pain in my ear.

The medical doctors didn't see anything in my ears, because there was nothing wrong with my ears.

So I started getting adjusted. Soon after, I stopped getting the episodes of ear pain. I said, "Wow, I move better! Wow, I have an answer for what was wrong with me!"

The chiropractor said, "I don't do anything except restore the body back to its proper alignment and balance. That lets the nerves communicate properly."

That fast, I was fascinated with chiropractic.

Throughout the rest of high school, I enjoyed studying health and science. Then I thought, "Hm. My cousin is going to be a pharmacist. Pharmacists make good money." With that in mind, I started a pre-pharmacy major in college.

Then one day I walked into a chiropractic office in need of an adjustment. I knew I didn't feel right and knew he could help me. I went in, and he said, "Hey, do you want a job?"

At the time I was working at Walmart. I thought, "*Walmart associate* verses *chiropractic assistant* on a resume. That looks a lot better for college applications and future jobs." I answered, "Yeah! Sounds great!"

I didn't really think about it being a long-term career, but for six months I worked there and observed the chiropractor. I held the chart for him and preformed therapy for him. I saw the same kind of experience I'd had when I was twelve. People came in who didn't have things going right, and they'd leave doing better and recovering.

And I thought, "This is pretty cool."

The chiropractor told me I should become a chiropractor. But when you're a freshman in college, nobody's going to tell you what to do because "we know better!" I mentally shrugged and thought, "Okay, whatever."

The job was only a temporary position. He was holding it for someone else. After six months, I went back to a retail job.

Now during the months I worked for the chiropractor, my primary medical doctor, who had referred me to the chiropractor, came in for a couple of treatments. While working retail again, I developed a sinus infection. So I went to see the medical doctor.

He said, "Hey, are you still working for the chiropractor?"

I said, "No, it was a temporary position."

"Oh? I have a receptionist's job available. Are you interested?"

"Yes!"

During that job working for the medical doctor, I started truly seeing the division, the difference, between allopathic and holistic medicine. This medical doctor was very open-minded to chiropractic and acupuncture. He also recommended some healthy supplements and shakes to his patients, and he did a few more evaluations than most MDs.

While I work at the office, drug representatives came and fed us lunch three days a week—to the doctor, the staff, and me—and presented their in-house-generated (biased) reports about why patients should take their drugs.

After they left, I began seeing a trend, that of the doctor and medical staff being influenced. Based on the drug reps' sales tactics, they were thinking, "These reports that the drug reps are presenting should be true, right? Because, it's a study and also they were nice and gave us a delicious lunch."

I also saw the trend of people coming in who were sick, and they'd be put on a drug that didn't work, so they'd go on another drug, or they'd have a side effect and have to take another drug to mask the side effects of that drug.

And I noticed that the pharmacist, what I had thought I wanted to be, was a middleman. We'd call in scripts from the doctor, and the pharmacist would fill them. Then when patients would go to the pharmacist, the pharmacist would say, "Take these with food; $10 copay." Pharmacists had phenomenal knowledge, but they were the middleman. They didn't problem-solve. I realized I wanted to help problem-solve. I wanted to help these people evolve and not just Band-Aid their illnesses.

The chiropractor I had worked for, I recalled, had helped patients to actually heal. When people came in, they got better. There was no side effect. There was a little initial soreness, but patients continued to evolve and get better. Whereas these people who came to see the medical doctor were stuck. All they did was take drugs. However, the people he did treat with some of the holistic foods and supplements did get better.

I decided, "No, I don't want to be a pharmacist. It's at the chiropractor's office that people evolve and heal."

It was a divine path, because I literally walked into places and miraculously the doors just opened. "Hey, you want a job?"

"Okay! Sounds good."

Chiropractic office. Medical doctor office. I saw people get better. I saw people not get better.

I thought, "You know what? I want to be a chiropractor."

That's where my chiropractic and health journey started, and led to where I am today. I found my passion for nutrition and vibrant living.

I love to see people thrive. I love people overcoming physical obstacles, or relationship obstacles, or any kind of obstacle. I love to see people grow and reach their full potential.

That's my vision—I want to see people have optimal health. I want to help them—help *you*—get the best out of your body that you can.

I never want you to settle for unhealthy-normal.

Are you ready to leave unhealthy behind? Then turn the page, and take your first step toward a new normal.

A healthy, vibrant you awaits!

℞ **Health** is vibrant physical, mental, social, and spiritual functioning and well-being. Not just the absence of symptoms or disease.

Your Body:
OWNERS ~ Investments That Pay Off

It seems everybody is worried about investing in their retirement these days. We realize the government may not be able to sustain us and that Medicare could go away. So, we try to stash money away so we have money for later.

What about the investment in our bodies? Day after day we fill our bodies with junk foods and non-foods, and we heap ourselves with mental stresses. When we get to the point of retirement, much of the money we put away is going to be used up trying to keep us healthy. It'll go to drug companies because we didn't invest in our health.

It's time to take a stand and say, "I want to be healthy *now*."

That's why you picked up this book. You've made the choice to invest in your health.

So how will you invest?

To determine that, you first need to know what you want your future to look like healthwise.

The Future You

Here's a mental exercise many find highly beneficial. Ask yourself, "What kind of life do I want years from now?" "What kind of health and body do I want to have?"

Take time and really consider this. Let yourself fully envision the future you.

Do you want to be able to play with your grandkids when you're in your sixties? Golf in your seventies? Travel in your eighties?

What do you want to feel like short-term and long-term? Short-term might be getting more energy, feeling more active. Long-term might be having your tissues, organs, and cells working efficiently.

Think about those things. Prioritize those things.

Whatever you focus on and work toward you can achieve.

(Within reason and possible reality. If you're four-foot-one, you're probably not going to be a basketball star. You're not going to be able to do certain things. But also it was Walt Disney who said, "It's kinda fun to do the impossible.")

Once you've decided what you want your future to look like healthwise, evaluate your health as it is today.

Assess Your Current Health

Everything about your body is interconnected. And anytime you overload any system, it can cause illness.

Symptoms are your body trying to tell you something. Pain has purpose. If you have symptoms or pain, it's because there's an *underlying* problem.

Symptoms are not the disease. They are the flares that signal something else is wrong.

My focus is on health, not on disease. I don't want to label your disease. I don't want to label you with chronic fatigue, and I don't want to label you with diabetes. When you aren't feeling well, that is a symptom. Chronic fatigue and diabetes are just symptoms of the gut, pancreas, liver, or brain not functioning optimally.

If you're not feeling well, I want to focus on, "Okay, what can we improve?"

You don't have to accept the labels and limits that are put on us. "It's arthritis. I just have to live with the pain." Or, "I can't play sports anymore."

No, often that's not what it is. You don't have to live in pain. We can eliminate those symptoms—not just mask them—and live a healthier life.

So what are your current symptoms? What do you need to improve healthwise in order to move toward the vibrant, future you?

Take a few minutes and list any occasional or chronic symptoms here.

_____

_____

_____

_____

Now you know where you are and where you're going—the future you. You know what you're investing in. In the weeks ahead, you can come back and track your progress.

Direct Your Focus

I compare health to light. And I compare disease and dysfunction to darkness. If we increase light, then darkness decreases.

Think of it this way. When you walk into a dark room, you focus on increasing the light, not trying to get rid of the darkness. The darkness goes away easily when you simply increase the light.

Likewise, when we are health-focused, then our health improves. But when neglect our health, disease and dysfunction increase.

Our society is focused on disease and dysfunction. As a result, we have more disease and dysfunction. If instead we focus on health, we will have a different result. We will have improvement in health.

We need to re-direct our focus.

Make a conscious effort to focus on health by asking, "What kind of things can I do to make my body function more optimally?"

Disease <-------USA--------- | ----------------------> Health

We have two sides to the spectrum. Your health is on one end. Disease is on the other. Some people choose to ignore symptoms until the disease is too much for them to bear . . . or when it's too late to reverse the causes of the problem. That's true whether we are speaking of the physical body or other aspects of life.

There are always consequences when we don't listen to the earliest signs of problems. The cancer or the disease just didn't happen overnight.

So direct your focus. What's going to move you in the direction toward health? What steps are you going to take to get moving that way?

The good news is that your body is doing most of the work already! Your body is overcoming the odds right now, keeping you alive despite our society's toxic eating habits and environment.

It's stunning how many chemical reactions and other operations go on automatically in our body, on a regular basis. Even when you're not feeling well, your body is still working and doing all those processes.

The miracle of the body is that it is wise, and it knows how to regulate things. It just needs a little more help from you.

It's like when you buy an older classic car. You can tweak things. You can put better gas in it. You can make sure the oil is changed regularly. You can get the car running as optimally as possible.

The car is intact. It's still there. You can enhance it. You still see many classic cars on the roads these days because their owners took care of them and the creator of those cars made them to last, our bodies were made to last.

Our bodies' foundation is strong. The DNA is in there. Everything we need is in there. Our bodies are designed to heal themselves. We just need to give our bodies what they need to function optimally. That's where you have to put in the effort.

If we just abuse the car and keep abusing it, then yeah, we're not going to see any positive changes. There is an effort. But once you start making those changes, you start to see, "Oh, wow. The car's going faster. It's not as loud. Now it runs smooth. This baby is awesome!"

Same concept, right? We have to invest in ourselves.

We can't leave the care of our health to just doctors. We are the OWNERS of our bodies.

The acronym OWNERS reminds us what we need to give our bodies so they can heal themselves:

- ☒ **O**xygen
- ☒ **W**ater
- ☒ **N**utrients
- ☒ **E**xercise
- ☒ **R**est
- ☒ **S**ocial and Spiritual Health

Investing in those is what will eliminate symptoms of illness. Those are the investments that will pay off.

The Big Picture

As I've said, we are designed to be healthy. The problem is that we are bombarded in a society of stresses—physically, mental, psychological, and emotional.

For example, **oxygen**. We have things in our air that we didn't have before, and not only pollutants. No one thinks about it. They're excited when we get, "Oh! Free Wi-Fi!" But we don't yet know what all these wavelengths are doing when they pass through our bodies. That research has not been done. We don't know how that might be affecting us on a cellular level or energetic level.

Water. Pesticides from farm fields and weed-free chem lawns get into well water. Tap water often contains heavy metals and chemicals, whether city water or well water. Unhealthy water stresses the body.

Nutrients. In our physical environments, we have nonfood in our food. Our food is now heavily polluted with pesticides, antibiotics, hormones, and other nonfoods—such as preservatives, artificial colorings, and artificial flavorings.

Food should be fuel and energy. All that extra stuff should not be in there. And when you put all that extra stuff in there, that's a stress on the body, because the body then has to deal with those extras and eliminate them, because they're not useful but harmful. In many respects, not only is food not fuel and energy like it should be, it's anti-fuel and anti-energy.

Amazingly, many people don't even realize it. We're conditioned since childhood with books and advertising to believe what we're told. We don't stop and think anymore, or take time to be mindful of what we're doing. We need to wake up! Think, "What am I putting into my body?"

Exercise. If we are not at our optimal condition, if we have to struggle physically, then our physical stress can lead to mental and emotional stress.

It's as if we have a resource bank. If we take care of our bodies physically, then we have more resources to deal with the other aspects of our lives. If we don't exercise, we lose those resources.

Rest. In our fast-paced, blitz-through-life society, almost no one gets enough rest. We pack kids' schedules tight with school and year-round extracurricular activities. We pack our own schedules with so much work we wish we could be cloned. We even pack our weekends and vacations with activities. Few people rest. Many people develop diseases because of this.

Social health. In our society, we have less structure in our families, and that affects us emotionally. Children are dealing with more as divorce rates keep going up. They have to deal with changing dynamics, because now they not only have one unit of family, but now they have two or more family units. They have to try to figure out those challenges in their home lives.

And we have a lot more mental stresses for the same reasons as well as with work, especially since the economy isn't really predictable. We have little time for family. Little time for friendships. Little time for the relationships we need to fulfill us.

As a society, we have more and more psychological issues.

Spiritual health. We have no time to meditate, to center ourselves. We spend what little free time we have on electronic devices. We don't go for walks in nature. We don't refresh our spirits.

That's the big picture. And that's what we're going to address. How? By taking OWNERShip.

Say, "Hey, I have a choice. I know I have this history physically, mentally, or emotionally, but I have a choice of how I respond from now on. Today I can take ownership of my choices.

"I can make a choice to stop buying and ingesting destructive foods. No more. I'm not going to eat sugars or go for the sweets. I'm going to make better choices picking fruits and vegetables that I can handle. I'm going to say no to so much adrenal-taxing coffee and yes to more nourishing, hydrating water.

"I have a choice to have boundaries in what I tolerate in my home or at work." If you have an abusive boss or coworker, you have a choice to say, "No, I'm not going to let you treat me like this," and stand up for yourself in those aspects, and make those social boundaries.

You also have a choice to take evaluation of your life and say, "Where do I need help? What am I not capable of correcting on my own? Where do I need to seek a wellness professional who can assist me in making these changes that I can't do myself?"

Maybe you would even benefit from help in evaluating your physical, mental, and emotional health. Simply step up and say, "I know there's something not right. I'm not healthy, and this is not healthy. I need to be proactive and make a change." There are many resources out there. You can go through a health check list online or go to a library and find many books on this. If you want someone else to evaluate and help you, look up a local wellness chiropractor and/or holistic doctor to help you identify where you can improve your health and make positive changes.

We're going to keep it simple. While you read the chapters ahead, we'll take a look at your physical, mental, and emotional health, then you can just begin to change one or two things. In time you can go back and change more. But start with, "Here is a variety of things I could begin to work on." Read the chapters, pick what's talking to you the most right now, and then go from there. Later you can come back to the book and try something else, and keep going through it.

Some people have personalities that are all or nothing. They'll try to tackle the whole thing, every health issue they need to change. If that is you, God bless you! That's just fine if that is what works for you. But most people I know gain the most success from taking one step at a time. You get a little bit closer, and a little bit closer, and your progress inspires you. You keep going. For most people it's wise not to take on so much that steps become gigantic and overwhelming.

That's how I deal with my patients. I have patients who come in, and if they're drinking a pack of soda or a pot of coffee a day, I'm not going to expect them to give up that whole thing all at once. I say, "Okay, let's do one less." And the next time, "Let's do another one less." Then, "Can you switch two of those with a glass of water?" And generally patients will back down on their sugar or caffeine intake over time.

I have few patients who say, "Forget it! I'm done with sugar or caffeine. I've seen what it does to me!" And they throw out all their remaining soda or coffee, just like that.

But the majority of patients are not that way. The majority of people just work their way into the new habit.

When you take steps to improve your health, avoid being rigid with yourself. Instead, take easy steps! One of my patients recently started a purification protocol. After a few days she said, "Oh my goodness, all these supplements. I cannot do this. Is there another way?"

I said, "If there are too many to swallow, let's cut the dose in half. You'll still get some benefits. If you can't choke them down, what's the point? You're not going to get any benefit at all if you quit."

Take baby steps. What can you do to move yourself even a little bit toward more vibrant health? I don't want you to give up and make the mountain so high that you can't get there. I want you to say, "Okay, what baby step can I do? What small thing can I change?"

I don't like rigidness. I like people to be able to be flexible. Goals should help set you free not chain you down.

If you're a goal-setter, set SMART goals for yourself. Goals should be:

- Specific
- Measurable
- Achievable
- Realistic
- Timely (There's no unreasonable goals, just unreasonable time frames. If you put yourself in a ten-year goal and try to accomplish it in one year, then you set yourself up for failure.)

Whatever works for you, just get that ball rolling in the right direction. Keep things easy!

Right about now, you might be wondering, "How long will it take before I start feeling better and recovering from some of my illnesses?"

Generally it takes a month to three months to see that your health is improving. One month if you have just a few or light symptoms, and closer to three months if you're dealing with more symptoms.

That is, as long as you're following through as consistently as possible, if you're making the changes and taking responsibility for them.

A lot of times patients come in to my office and say, "I don't feel better."

I ask, "Well, are you following the diet?"

And they say, "No. . . ."

Then I say, "Well, you can't blame it on my advice if you're not doing it. You have to follow through."

When you follow through, you're going to see changes. Once we start respecting our bodies, it's amazing how quickly positive changes happen. Clearer thinking. More energy. Some weight loss.

I don't really focus on weight loss. I just focus on vitality. That's it. Just overall vitality.

That being said, people with chronic diseases such as diabetes benefit with a changed diet and see positive improvements.

And when you take small, simple advancements, follow-through is easier.

Oxygen:
You Are What You Breathe

We are OWNERS of our bodies. For your first step toward vibrant health, we'll focus on oxygen.

How?

First, make sure you are breathing. Partially inflated lungs isn't breathing! So many patients come in to my office who I'll ask to take a deep breath, and they don't know what that is! So, I actually have them practice drawing deep breaths in. I have them take plenty of time to sit up nice and tall, shoulders back, and just fill their lungs deeply, four times.

When they leave I tell them, "I want you to do that two times a day. Have a little alarm that reminds you, and then sit up, put your shoulders back to open your lungs, and take four nice, deep breaths. Breathe all the way in, visualizing your lungs being balloons, and fill them all the way down using the diaphragm muscle (the muscle at the bottom of your ribcage). *Really* breathe and bring up your oxygen levels."

Four deep breaths twice a day—that alone can destress you a little, because it shifts your autonomic nervous system into rest-and-digest mode. It floods your brain cells with more oxygen. It also helps clear your mind a bit, because you're focused on the breathing.

People talk about counting to ten when you get mad. That's smart, but also take those four deep, calming, cleansing breaths works too.

ᛞ Take OWNERShip—Oxygen

If you want to take this step toward more vibrant health . . .

- ✓ For the next several moments, practice breathing deeply. Sit up, put your shoulders back to open your lungs, and take four nice, deep breaths. Breathe all the way in, visualizing your lungs being balloons, and fill them all the way down with the diaphragm. Hold for the count of 4 to 6. Release air slowly.
- ✓ Set an alarm to remind yourself to enjoy four deep breaths twice a day.

Oxygen also has to do with the *quality* of air you breathe, the physical aspects of oxygen.

Evaluate your home and workplace. Are you taking the proper precautions to make sure you aren't breathing in chemicals and pollutants? Why does this matter? Because almost everything we breathe gets a direct line to our blood system. Whatever quality of oxygen we breathe goes straight into our blood.

We have more chemicals in our households, under our kitchen sinks, than chemists in the 1940s had in their labs! We have easy access to all these chemicals nowadays, and that is polluting our households and the places we work.

So you want to try to eliminate as many chemicals and pollutants in the home and workplace as possible. Try to go with some of the natural, Earth-friendly green cleaners. Research brand recommendations on the Internet.

You can also use baking soda (old baking soda from your fridge or freezer makes a great cleaner!). You can use vinegar. Both work very well.

Be sure to switch to a natural, Earth-friendly laundry detergent. The laundry detergent aisle at the grocery store is usually the strongest smelling aisle. That's because the chemical scents seep through the plastic bottles. Then we breathe those chemicals.

Breathing chemicals is true of scented candles too. Candle manufacturers put a *lot* of chemicals in candles. Candle wax—paraffin wax—is made from bleaching and deodorizing petroleum waste. And when you burn the candles, those chemicals get released into the air.

Benzene and toluene (which are carcinogens) are a few of the chemicals released by burning the base wax alone. The wicks? About 30 percent of candle wicks are made with heavy metals, such as lead.

Most scented candles produce soot and smoke equivalent to those you'd breathe if you were sitting in front of a diesel engine.

Plug-in room scents also contain pollutants. We want our homes to smell good, but we don't think about all those chemicals that get released. Some people get headaches from those chemical smells.

Instead, we could simply boil cinnamon in a little pot of water and make the home smell cinnamon-y. That way we get the good smells, without the chemicals. You could also defuse essential oils.

Don't get me wrong—there are good companies that don't add chemicals, products that are more natural, but you need to search for those.

There are a lot of essential oils that you can buy that don't pollute the oxygen you breathe. Essential oils can also lift or enhance your mood. A quick online search will give you some great ideas of essential oils to try.

Also, have your home tested for radon gas. In seven states that were studied, about one in three homes had unsafe levels of radon gas. Long-term exposure causes lung cancer.

Make these simple changes to create an environment that gives you plenty of good, clean oxygen.

What you breathe directly affects your health.

℞ Take OWNERShip—Oxygen

If you want to take this step toward more vibrant health . . .

✓ In your home and workplace, try to exchange chemicals for green cleaners and detergents.
✓ Exchange candles and plug-in room scents for mood-enhancing essential oils, or boil a pot of cinnamon water.
✓ Test your home for radon gas. Mitigate if needed.

ᘯ Four

Want Vitality?
Water *Works!*

A majority of your body is water—the W in OWNERS.

Water is your overall solvent.

So you need to make sure you have a good, steady supply to help you sparkle.

If you think about it, your bodies like a fish tank. If you're not putting water in and cleaning out the tank, it's going to be gross! The crud is just going to accumulate.

How Much?

So how much water should you drink? I pretty much go with the old standard. If you can get in eight glasses, you're doing a good job!

As always, keep it simple. If you can't drink eight glasses, drink what you can. Even a little more than you normally drink is better.

If you can only increase your intake by a glassful a day each month, and you slowly work your way up to seven or eight glasses a day over time, great!

Change is often easier and longer lasting if you do a little at a time.

Water, or *Fluid*?

A frequent comment I get from patients is, "Well, I drink coffee, tea, or soda, it has water in it, so it's water."

I explain, "No, it has to be water. Straight water."

People say, "But I don't like the taste of water," or, "It's too boring."

I say, "Okay, you can add a little bit of lemon juice, or put in a slice of cucumber or ginger. But you need to try to get as much straight water as you can. Just get up to those eight glasses. On a regular basis."

(In case you haven't guessed, I'm saying this to you too.)

Coffee, tea and soda have caffeine, a diarrheic. Even decaffeinated coffee has some caffeine in it; it's not completely caffeine-free. Caffeine affects the kidneys to stop holding back water by interfering with a hormone called ADH anti diuretic hormone. So for every cup of caffeinated coffee or tea you drink, you now have that caffeine revving your adrenaline, which also increases your blood sugar since your body thinks you're in fight-or-flight mode, and you have other chemicals that the body has to try to get rid of. And you're actually dehydrating yourself.

So for every cup of caffeinated coffee or tea you drink, you need to drink a glass of water just to counteract the dehydration. Then you need another glass to start hydrating yourself.

If you drink two cups of coffee, then your body will need four glasses of water.

More Q & A

People tell me, "Well, I've gone without drinking all that water for years."

I explain, "Yes, and you've stressed your body with it." Your body does what it needs to do because it's amazing and adaptable. But insufficient hydration stresses your body. That stress depletes your energy.

A lack of hydration depletes your energy too. So does the lack of oxygen that your body and brain aren't getting.

Then people say, "Well, I have to pee more when I drink water."

I reply, "For a while, you will, yes, until your body adapts." You have to give your body time to get used to it, because it's not used to drinking all this water. And now your body thinks, "Wow, they're actually giving it to me. What am I supposed to do with this? Am I going to get more?"

But when you continually do drink enough water, then your body will start to adapt and regenerate. It'll think, "Oh, now I'm getting what I need! Great! Let's filter you out." It takes a while before the body actually starts the cleaning process. So at first you'll pee more, and that's the start of something good.

If people increase their water intake and say, "It's still going through me, Doc," then I tell them, "The water isn't taking hold because your body is lacking minerals. So add about half a teaspoon of sea salt (Celtic or Himalayan) to your water each day." It works!

Occasionally I get the question of, "Can a person overdrink water?"

I think that a few years ago some evil parent made their daughter drink gallons of water, and the girl died. It's rare; you actually have to be in that situation where you're forcing someone to drink, drink, drink. It's very rare that overdrinking water causes an issue.

Usually your body tells you to stop. "Okay, I'm good."

Someone might say, "Well, if the body tells you what it needs, and you're not feeling thirsty, then why would you drink when you're not thirsty?"

If you've ignored or corrupted your body, it's desensitized. It doesn't know what it needs. A lot of people are desensitized to thirst. Because they've ignored the body, the body's no longer saying, "You need water." It's learned it has to function less because it has had less.

Give your body what it needs.

Water Testing and Filtration

Tap water often contains chemicals and heavy metals, whether it's city water or well water.

Is your tap water clean? If you're not certain, have your water tested. A lot of communities have organizations that test your water sample. Be sure to test for heavy metals and chemicals.

Do you have bacteria in your water? Or in your pipes? I've heard stories of people who had bacterial buildup in their pipes, but they didn't know it until they became ill. A filtration system on the faucet or in the fridge will pull out some of that, but not all. Plus, you're showering in it. You don't think about it, but showering still exposes you to that bacteria. The water splashes in your face—eyes, nose, mouth, and ears.

We get a report from my local community, and it indicates, "You have this and this in your water, but they're at acceptable levels."

My response is, "Acceptable levels! Really?? Zero is an acceptable level for me!"

If you're not able to test, or if your test results are grim, buy gallons of spring water or distilled water to drink.

Why spring water? Read on!

Drinking Water

Mostly I'm happy when people get enough water in, but it's also important to drink the healthiest water.

Most bottled water is tap water, even the water sold by big-name companies. It's the tap water of wherever it's bottled. It's likely not any cleaner than your tap water.

So that's where you've got to be careful. Read those labels. If it says "packaged in New York," it's New York tap water. You might as well just drink your own tap water instead of drinking that.

Just make sure your drinking water is clean. Use a reverse osmosis filtration system if you want to be certain. With RO water, you can add a little sea salt into it to get some electrolytes back and at the same time be confident that you have no pollutants in what you are drinking.

If you're going to do bottled, spring water should have natural minerals and electrolytes in it. This would make it the best to purchase.

About Plastic Bottles

Water bottles are made of toxic plastics, which is another problem, since the mouth and digestive juices touch the plastic when people drink from individual bottles.

The toxins from plastics can go in our bodies and act negatively on our cells. And some of them can activate and throw off hormones, called xenohormones or xenoestrogens. These can cause fertility issues as well as cancer, and have also been linked to diabetes and heart disease.

The recycle number in the small triangles on bottles should be four or above. Five is even better. Avoid one through three.

The higher the number, the *thicker and better* the plastic, and the less residue it will leave in the water or in any food you buy that is packaged in plastic. The less toxic it will be.

When you see "fifty percent less plastic," usually that's a sign that the plastic is thinner and more toxic.

Thinner plastics are more degradable, especially in extreme temperatures, so they'll dissolve more into your drinking water or packaged food.

You've drunk plastic before if you left a water bottle in a hot car then had a sip. The water tastes like plastic tea.

With less plastics, okay, we're helping the environment, but are the toxins we consume worth it?

A lot of people have begun carrying around glass bottles enclosed in rubber, so if the bottle drops, it doesn't shatter. These glass bottles are commonly sold at retail stores. People are switching to glass because they want to get the plastic out of what they're drinking.

So nourish and refresh yourself with natural spring water, and drink from a glass or a ceramic cup or mug.

Most importantly, get that water in!

ᛉ Take OWNERShip—Water

If you want to take this step toward more vibrant health . . .

✓ Good hydration gives you energy! Try drinking more water. Eight glasses a day will do wonders, but even a little more than you normally drink will be beneficial.

✓ You can add a little lemon juice or a slice of cucumber or ginger. But you need to try to get as much straight water as you can.

✓ Is your tap water clean? If you're not certain, have your water tested, especially for heavy metals and bacteria.

✓ If you can, replace your plastic drinking bottles with glass. If you prefer plastic, try to stick with recycle numbers four and above. They're thicker plastic, so they're less toxic. Avoid one through three and anything that says "fifty percent less plastic."

Nutrients:
Some Unexpected Insights

We've arrived at the next letter in OWNERS—N. Nutrition.

There are a number of reasons why a body can't heal. Here are four of the most common ones.

- Communication is not happening. The brain and rest of the nervous system, the nervous system impulses, aren't communicating, so the body doesn't have control over, or understanding of, what's going on.
- Communication is not happening in the endocrine system—the chemical messengers. There's some malfunction going on, some interference in there.
- Inflammation. Due to a culture of high stress and toxic foods and environments, your immune system could be on overload and highly reactive. Your immune system may be targeting some of the things you eat, resulting in ongoing food sensitivities and inflaming your gut.
- The proper building blocks—nutrients—aren't being put into your body through right food choices.

Consider that fourth reason. With our Standard American Diet (SAD), we're not truly feeding ourselves. We're not giving the body the nutrients it needs to function the way it was designed.

Most people eat food for only one purpose: so that the stomach stops feeling hungry. But food shouldn't just fill the stomach. It has to be rich in the vitamins and minerals that feed and fuel your cells. Only then can your body heal itself and give you energy.

If you're lacking nutrients, your body is going to struggle. Your body can't regenerate your liver, skin or other organs out of nothing. You have to feed your body with the nutrients it requires.

Building Blocks

We think we're a solid unit, but we're not. All cells in the human body are turned over every seven years. Every single cell in our body is turned over. So, what are we, then?

Think back. You have the body now that you started nourishing seven years ago. You are what you have eaten.

However, our skin turns over more quickly. So does our gut lining.

If we start putting in the right foods and nutrients now and remove the interferences that are in our systems, we are going to have some more immediate results. We don't have to wait seven years for that.

Nutrition is not just about you. You're feeding your future.

If you research indigenous tribes, you'll find that many tribes feed pregnant women the best foods. They take care of the next generation. Our society often thinks, "Because you're pregnant, eat what you want." It's a different way of thinking. One group invests in the future, while the other focuses on the pleasure of what you want to eat now, and our children are developing more and more health issues.

(You can read more about indigenous tribes and the generational results of healthy eating habits in the book *The Blue Zones: Lessons for Living Longer From the People Who've Lived the Longest* by Dan Buettner, published by National Geographic.)

When Building Blocks Become Wrecking Balls: Manufactured Foods

Ninety years ago, only about 20 percent of the food people ate was processed. Today, only 10 percent of food is not processed. We totally went in the opposite direction of what our grandparents did. They are living into their nineties, and some are over a hundred years old.

My oldest patient recently passed away at 102 years of age, but that generation had a different start, a healthier way of eating for their first several decades.

The food industry has changed drastically. That is a reason why so many people suffer from illnesses.

Research came out a couple years ago that shows our children are not predicted to live as long as we are because of the way the trends are going, with our foods becoming more and more unhealthy and our disease rate climbing. We're already seeing the next generation's lifespans shortening because of these trends.

Many researchers see the trend, but they're not saying the *why*. One why is, obviously, that around 90 percent of the food we're eating is highly processed. And we're eating more processed sugar and non-foods.

Only a hundred years ago, each person ate, on average, just a pound of sugar a year. Today we're each averaging a pound of sugar or more a week. Not to mention, all the sugar-like additives.

It's ridiculous, how much sugar we are putting in. We are stressing our bodies to the max. (That's another testament to how amazing the body is, that our bodies haven't totally given up on us, with how much we're stressing them.)

I've trained my kids to read the cereal boxes. When they used to go in the cereal aisle, they'd grab a box and say, "I want this cereal."

I would reply, "Okay, if you can find one under six grams of sugar per serving (one and a half teaspoons per cup of cereal), you can get it."

They'd look at the label and say, "Uh, this one has twenty grams of sugar, Mom!"

Exactly. I taught my kids young. I call it garbage cereal. It's funny. The kids will go to our relatives then come home and say, "I had garbage cereal, Mom, while I was over there."

I respond, "I'm glad you enjoyed it over there." I don't say, "I'll not let you have anything unhealthy," because they'll binge eat after they are grown or out of my home and they're out on their own. I want them to feel and understand the difference of healthy food vs. unhealthy food for themselves.

Sugar-infusion doesn't end with breakfast cereal. It's in almost everything, including savory canned soups, macaroni and cheese . . . things you'd never even think to add sugar to if you made the food at home.

What about the chickens today? During processing most of them are injected with corn syrup or sugar. They're now sugar chickens! Food producers do this because we're a sugar-addicted society. They want to keep the consumer coming back. Is it any wonder so many people are becoming diabetics? Be sure to read every label to see whether the chicken you're holding contains sugars. It's crazy!

Even iodized sea salt contains sugar, because sugar is a flavor enhancer.

Food manufacturers add artificial coloring, flavorings, and flavor enhancers. All of these flavorings are chemically designed to enhance the taste process so that you like what you eat.

Oreos are engineered, on purpose, to contain *every* flavor enhancer that lights up the brain. That's why people can't sit and eat one Oreo. They want to eat the whole package.

Does a box or package announce "New and Improved!"? That usually means the manufacturer didn't improve it—as in, make it healthier—but that they added something artificial, such as flavorings to affect how your brain responds to it. Whenever they say "New and Improved!" they shifted something.

The food or beverage might be something you buy often, and then and all of a sudden you taste it and think, "Whoa, whoa, whoa! What happened?"

Food manufacturers also add preservatives so those items can stay on the shelf longer. *Years* longer.

Consider this. Each of our bodies is constantly producing cancer cells. Everybody, everyday has cancer cells that are produced in their body. With some people it turns into a huge mass. But with most healthy people, the body goes, "Hey! That's an abnormal cell! Tag it! Destroy it! Get rid of it!" The body recognizes it and keeps the body healthy.

However, some people's immune systems get distracted by all the other junk that's in the body, and by stresses. The immune system is so busy cleaning up that it doesn't have time to recognize this other abnormal cell. So the cancer cell grows and spreads.

When we start eliminating junky, processed food and stress, that frees up the body to be healthier.

A ten-year study was done on women nurses who ate a diet rich in fruits and vegetables. They had fewer incidences of cancer, diabetes, and weight issues. It's because they didn't have the physical and mental stresses on them caused by a junky diet. The body was able to function properly and heal itself.

How does the medical field usually handle this?

What unfortunately happens often in medical doctors' offices is they tell patients, "Yes, you should eat better, but here's a drug that'll control your sugars." That doctor might send patients to a dietician, but a lot of times the dieticians' patients tell me that the dietician said, "Oh, diet soda's okay! You can do diet soda." *Grr!*

These are medical dieticians, so they're not really focused on healing the underlying problem or on how natural our bodies were designed to be. They say, "Yeah, you should eat more vegetables, and don't eat a lot of cookies and candies, but it's okay to do the 'diet' or the 'sugar-free' stuff."

It *isn't* okay! Diet and sugar-free stuff is just as bad on the liver and harmful to many other parts of your body. Those are nonfoods!

Dieticians should say, "No, you need to eat cleaner foods."

So a lot of times when patients come to me with health issues while feeding themselves junk food, I have no tolerance for those foods. They're not beneficial to the body at all. If patients try to make excuses for eating junk food and I see them so unhealthy, I even get mad. I say, "No! It's not simply junk food. It's a neural toxin! Go look it up on the internet!"

Not even ants will go near diet soda that's been spilled. And that's what I tell people! No self-respecting insect or animal or bacteria will eat it! If nature will not touch the stuff, that means we should not be eating it!

We really are what we eat. If we keep eating junky, we'll keep feeling junky.

Eliminate your sugars. Go back to clean eating. Steer clear of processed foods.

If you read the label and don't recognize something as a food, or if you see a chemical or you can't pronounce a word, then that's usually not a good sign. That's extra junk your body has to process, that your body has to deal with and eliminate. That causes more stress on the body.

So if the package says it's carrot sticks, then the label should read *carrots, water*. Canned beets should be just *beets* and *water*. But even many canned beets will contain high fructose corn syrup. Really!? They took a healthy vegetable and added corn syrup?

The processed food industry is not about health. It's about selling products, particularly products that are addictive.

On my vision board, I've posted Gandhi's Seven Social Sins. One is "commerce without morality." People must have a moral center, or they don't deserve our trust *or* our business. But in the processed food industry, commerce is all about producing money. It's just not good.

Gandhi's Seven Social Sins

Wealth without work.
Pleasure without conscience.
Knowledge without character.

Commerce without morality.
Science without humanity.
Worship without sacrifice.
Politics without principle.

We need to eat foods not messed with by man. If it looks just like it did on the plant, that's what our bodies need.

Manipulation

People think it's cool that some vegetables are being grown hydroponically, but nutrient-wise, a tomato produced that way is basically a red shell with water. Just water and red, little nutrients to speak of.

That can fill your stomach, but it won't adequately heal and fuel your body.

Will a car engine with no motor oil keep on running well?

Hydroponic growers add synthetic nutrients, which are not in the right state or form as those naturally found in good soil. That's technically not organic.

In addition, the growers raise these hydroponic foods in buildings like warehouses. They use lightbulbs, which means the foods have no real sun exposure. The sun is vastly different from the lights used in hydroponics. They're even different wavelengths.

Since I brought up the subject of technology as related to hydroponics, consider this: We have no idea how our technological devices, Wi-Fi, and microwave ovens are affecting us. We do know that microwaving your food denatures your vitamins, as opposed to warming it on the stove. It's wise to keep an eye out for articles that reveal the progress of research on these.

GMO stands for Genetically Modified Organism. GMO is another result of technology and human manipulation. Genetic modifying is manipulating nature. Essentially the scientists splice bacteria with plants. This allows the plants to grow in soil that is saturated with deadly pesticides.

When insects eat those plants, we know it makes their stomachs explode. What do you think that's doing to us?

I'll give you a hint. GMO foods also tear holes in the intestinal lining of bigger animals, such as squirrels, raccoons, and opossums that go into the cornfield, and the cows that eat the corn. Then we eat the GMO corn, and we eat the sick cows that ate the corn. (We also ingest the pesticides.) So GMO foods tear holes in the intestinal lining of animals. It does the same to us.

It's one way that results in what's known as leaky gut. Leaky gut is a foundation of bodily inflammation and autoimmune diseases.

We distort nature, but we do not know the long-term effects of it. When you create something new, just like a pharmaceutical drug, you don't know the long-term effects of it, because you're creating a new thing, a new product. It *is* a product because it's patented; it's no longer natural.

All the GMO foods man-made products that have we don't know all the ways the human body can react to them. This is seriously scary.

And that's the main concern. "We must be mindful of what we put into our bodies."

If you saw a berry you'd never seen before, would you pick it and eat it? Many berries are poisonous. If you don't know what kind of berry it is, are you going to put it in your mouth and swallow it? Or would you eat a mushroom you couldn't identify? Probably not, and berries and mushrooms are part of nature!

If we've created a GMO something and we're not really sure what we've created or what it might be doing to us, should we be putting it in our mouths?

As a culture, we're just manipulating nature left and right. And people are moving farther away from good, vibrant health.

Marketing

We live in an environment of sales, products, and marketing. That's part of our pursuit of happiness—to make a living from what we labor to create. But each time you hear any kind of marketing message, you need to weigh that message and not simply accept it. Ask yourself, "What all—good and bad—do consumers really get out of it?"

For example, mouthwash. The marketing message is, "You need mouthwash so that you can kiss your significant other or not offend your neighbors." You get a benefit, yes. You get fresh breath . . . for a few hours or so. But what's the long-term consequence of that?

Consider that mouthwash is antibacterial—it kills the bacteria (germs) that cause odors. However, our bodies are carefully balanced biomes of good bacteria, bad bacteria, yeasts, and other microorganisms, all of which, when correctly balanced, help the body break down foods, absorb nutrients, and stay healthy. When an antibacterial agent destroys bad bacteria, it also kills good bacteria, leaving room for the living microorganisms to take over and upset the natural, healthy balance.

The good and bad bacteria in the mouth are the first stage of digestion. When you kill off those bacteria, that stage of digestion doesn't take place, certainly not to the extent it needs to. That affects the rest of your digestive processes and how many nutrients your body will be able to break down and use! That's huge!

So, what can you do instead of using mouthwash? You can simply brush, floss, and rinse with a few drops of peppermint oil in water. It's simple, costs a lot less, and is much healthier. Coconut oil pulling is another option.

Before buying any "helpful" product you see advertised, always ask yourself, "But what's the long-term consequence of using this or eating this?"

If people have heartburn, they think that it's normal and they simply need antacids (for the rest of their lives, or at least for the foreseeable future). Since commercials bombard us with drugs that claim to reverse symptoms (temporarily), that makes consumers think, "Oh, I'm normal, because everybody else is getting antacids." And you think that's okay. It's become normal for our society, but a healthy body doesn't need antacids.

As a side note, acid reflux is usually caused by too *little* stomach acid. Good, strong stomach acid is needed to strengthen the lower esophageal aperture, the round door that keeps stomach acid from splashing up into the tender, sensitive tissues of the esophagus. Without enough stomach acid, that door becomes limp, and you experience acid reflux or "heartburn."

Acid reflux is a key symptom of an H. pylori bacterial infection in the stomach. H. pylori reduces your stomach's ability to make digestive acids and can never be cured by antacids. Even worse, antacids further nullify your natural digestive acids, making it even harder for your body to digest your food or draw healing nutrients from it.

Unfortunately, very few medical doctors test for or treat H. pylori. They simply prescribe an antacid "Band-Aid" to mask the symptoms so that you "feel fine" again.

Marketing. The United States is the only country that allows advertising to children of toys, cereal, and so on. Canada doesn't do it. Neither does Australia. Europeans will not. Why? Because children don't have the knowledge to filter truth. They see the marketing message and believe it has truth. They believe certain toys can fly, because that's what the commercials show—a toy car that goes airborne in an awesome feat of coolness. That's why the toys have little words on the bottom that kids can't read, "This product does not actually fly." But children want the toy because of the commercial or the cereal because its cartoon character spokesperson/creature spews enthusiastic messaging. Children trust the message as truth.

Even as adults we get fed marketing messages as truth. Drug manufacturers must now list side effects, but they do so quickly and often quietly or in small print, and all the while they've got this pretty butterfly on the screen trying to distract you along with energetic, happy people coming and going and living fabulous, fictionalized lives.

The last thing you'll hear is that the medication for depression causes depression and has been known to cause suicidal behavior.

"What's the long-term consequence of using or eating this?"

My family and I don't watch much TV, but I've trained my kids to evaluate these things. To their amusement, they've even heard me yell at commercials, "ARE YOU KIDDING ME!?"

They say, "Mom, it's a commercial, don't forget."

Yes, it is. But for consumers, it can have the effect of a wrecking ball.

The Real Origin of Healthier Skin

Consider your skin. Your skin is basically protein and oil. It's called the phospholipid layer—"phosphor" meaning protein, and "lipid" meaning fat. So, it's made with protein and fat.

Now, if you're not putting healthy protein and healthy fats into your body, yes, you're going to have acne. You're going to have dry skin.

If you're eating fake fats, you're going to have fake fat skin. If you're eating fast foods that are packed full of chemicals, that's what your skin's going to be like in the future. You'll have chemical skin.

When it comes to skin products, the general rule of thumb is this: If you can't eat it, then you shouldn't put it on your skin.

Why? Because your skin absorbs, and substances you put on can right into your body.

Think about it. Nicotine patches go on the skin to help a person stop smoking. Contraceptive patches go on the skin. So do hormone creams, estrogen creams. We know those things are absorbed by the skin, but we don't think about that on a daily basis, like when we put on an oil or a lotion. Be mindful. It's your body.

Even myself, I had never thought about the extent of what we absorb through the skin. Then one day a natural endocrinologist was talking about a male patient of hers. When she tested the patient to find out why he was having health issues, she found he had a certain hormone level that was very high. The natural endocrinologist helped him to discover the cause. The man's lotion that he liked because "it makes your skin soft" had trace hormones in it. That threw his hormone level off enough that he had to go to an endocrinologist. She had him stop using the lotion, and sure enough, his levels came back down. Simple things like that matter. With lotions, you've got to be careful.

Since we absorb whatever contacts our skin, start thinking about what you're exposed to. Are you a mechanic who is exposed to different greases and other substances? Make sure to protect yourself from that. Wear gloves when you can, and wash the stuff off as soon as you're able. If absorbed into your body, those things can cause toxic buildup. Whatever is in your environment comes through your skin.

And makeup as well. If you think about it, women wear makeup every day. Read every label. If a manufacturer won't tell you what's in the product, don't trust it. Their marketing says, "Oh, we're responsible. Our products are healthy. They're natural."

And I say, "Well, do you have XYZ in it? Any xenohormones?"

Their response? "We can't really tell you because it's patented, blah, blah, blah."

When they hide behind the legal aspect, then I don't trust them. If they won't reveal what's in a product, then I won't try it.

A lot of skin products have a mineral oil base. Mineral oil actually clogs the pours, so the products aren't doing our faces any good. Mineral oil, actually, is not good.

I've had people use olive oil for their skin, and coconut oil to remove their mascara. Products with real, natural oils or plant products for a base are also much better.

With skin products, again, look at the label. Are a bunch of chemicals listed? If you don't recognize half the things in it, then it's not that good for you. You want products that have the least amount of chemicals in them.

Today, some manufacturers are starting to move in a good direction with their skin products. You just need to read the labels.

How then do you get healthier skin? It goes back to nutrition. Eat healthy, nutrient-rich foods and healthy oils. Hydrate your skin by drinking plenty of good water. Hydration works from the inside out.

You can also visit a good health food store or shop online for nature-based alternatives.

Sunblocks and Lip Gloss—Are They Safe?

Most sunblocks contain oxybenzone (or benzophenone-3), and many of the –zones and –zines can lead to cancer. That means you're putting on sunblock so you don't get skin cancer, yet you're putting a chemical on your skin that can cause cancer! Oxybenzone also goes into makeup as a sunblock, so using that makeup can lead to cancer.

Instead, go with titanium dioxide and zinc oxides for your sunblocks. Those are the ones that are pasty and don't rub in very well, so you look pasty, but they don't have the possible negative results of the other sunblocks. Coconut oil has a SPF of 7. Cover up after 15 to 20 minutes, also wear a hat and don't let yourself get sunburned.

Have you thought about your lips? Some of my patients mention dry lips. "I'm addicted to that stuff that's supposed to heal chapped lips. Once I start wearing it, I feel like I have to keep wearing it."

Many manufacturers of lip gloss actually add an ingredient that makes your lips drier so you have to keep using the lip gloss. If you feel that your lips need balm often, that's likely why. Yet marketing tactics are designed to compel us to trust the companies to heal us.

At the office I have an olive-oil-based lip balm that works great. Many patients say, "Oh my goodness, it's the only chap stick I can use because of my chemical sensitivities."

"What's the long-term consequence of using or eating this?"

Bug Sprays are another thing you need to find a natural replacement for, essential oils are a better alternative.

Always, always ask that question before buying. Do your research. Uncover those unexpected insights.

Take OWNERShip of your body!

℞ Take OWNERShip—Nutrition

If you want to take this step toward more vibrant health . . .

- ✓ You have the body now that you started nourishing seven years ago. You are what you have eaten. If you haven't yet, start feeding your body more of the nutritious food it requires.
- ✓ Steer clear of processed foods, or at least read labels. Avoid the processed foods that contain sugar or have unknown ingredients.
- ✓ Choose organic.
- ✓ Avoid GMO foods.
- ✓ Instead of dangerous antibacterial mouthwash, acclimate to rinsing with a few drops of peppermint oil in water. Also, use ½ tablespoon of Virgin Organic Coconut oil by taking in the mouth, once melted swish for 5-10 minutes and spit out.
- ✓ If you use a lot of antacids to soothe your stomach, find a doctor who will test for H. pylori infection and be willing to actually cure it or find the cause of the symptom.
- ✓ Instead of using skin lotion packed with chemicals, visit a good health food store or shop online for nature-based alternatives.
- ✓ Use titanium dioxide and zinc oxides for your sunblocks.
- ✓ If lip balms aren't working, visit a good health food store or shop online for nature-based alternatives.

ॐ Six

Nutrients That Heal Your Body

Because nutrients and nutrition (OWNERS—N) are key to vibrant health, I've extended it to a second chapter.

In the previous chapter, we discovered unexpected insights about nutrition today, and some manufactured foods and products to avoid.

Now let's dig into the good stuff—the foods and nutrients we need to eat to heal our bodies . . . even from many chronic illnesses.

Advanced Organics

If we don't put good things into our bodies, then our bodies are not going to be able to produce the right product, in any situation. It's basic manufacturing. When you put good products put into something, you make a good-quality product at the end.

Do you eat substandard supplies? You're going to have a substandard product at the end. You're not going to have a fully strong product.

It's the same at our cellular level. If our cells aren't getting the nutrients they need and the vitamins that work the body's systems, then the body can't work or function properly. The body is great at doing what it can, but the body will not perform at its best.

Everyone knows we should eat fruits and vegetables, but the fruits and vegetables we are getting are severely nutrient-deficient. The soil has been over-cropped, it's not being replenished, and therefore the vegetables don't have much calcium, magnesium, or much of any base minerals. The vitamins are no longer enough there.

Look at what is good, better, and best. Try to eat and buy the best as you can.

And that means organic. Organic is best not only because it has fewer additives and fewer pesticides, but it's also much higher in nutrient content. Why? Because organic farmers make sure they're rotating crops and not depleting the soil.

If we can reach out and pluck it from an organic tree or plant, it's exponentially more nutrient-rich. It's so much better for us.

Several years ago, a study showed that an organic tomato had about sixteen hundred percent more iron than a hothouse tomato that was grown in very little soil. The study showed that organic had higher levels of all the nutrients we need—iron, calcium, and so on—verses commercially grown fruits and vegetables.

The closer to nature we can get, the more advanced the nutrition.

If man did *not* tamper with it, manipulate it, and package it, then it's what our bodies were designed to eat.

If you can grow your own garden, great! Hopefully that land has not been polluted with weed-killers and other substances. Hopefully it hasn't been over-cropped, so you'll be able to get as many nutrients as possible.

People are also doing community gardens. They lease out small spaces to have a neighborhood plot. That's a good trend you can look into. Even in cities people are trying to do rooftop gardens by getting good mineral-rich soil. There is Community Supported Agriculture (CSA) popping up all over the US too, see if one is near you.

So, eat nutrient-rich organic produce to begin healing your body.

And if you have a chronic illness, or long-term symptoms, that you want to be free of, the quickest way to start taking it down is with an elimination diet.

The Detoxifying, Health-Rejuvenating Elimination Diet

Symptoms are our bodies trying to tell us something. Pain has purpose. If you have symptoms or pain, it's because there's a problem.

A lot of people come in to my office and say, "I have pain in my joints. The medical doctor said I have arthritis and I just have to accept it."

I say, "Okay. At one time I had a ninety-nine-year-old patient. I know she had degeneration, because she was ninety-nine and bones wear down over time. They deteriorate. I'm not able to reverse that. But my ninety-nine-year-old patient had hip pain. After I adjusted her a couple of times, her pain was gone." Does that mean her arthritis was gone? I would say no, the body just wasn't adapting as well as it could have.

Degeneration and arthritis are *not* the same. And that's what medical doctors tend to say, "You have arthritis, which means you have degeneration." Not true! "-...itis" means inflammation. Arthritis is inflammation of the joint. We can eliminate inflammation by the foods we eat (and don't eat), which means we can eliminate the pain.

The pain is trying to tell you something. It's a signal.

You could be eating too much sugar. You might have a gluten sensitivity. You might be sensitive to food coloring.

Once you discover the catalyst, you can eliminate that food or substance, and then the inflammation—and the related pain or other related symptoms—will go away.

The illness or symptoms go away because that food has been eliminated, so your immune system is no longer reacting to it with inflammation. You have removed the cause.

Here is the elimination diet protocol that I use in my practice and highly recommend: the Standard Process 21-Day Purification Program (http://www.standardprocess.com/Standard-Process/Purification-Program#.VwatwkfdgoA). On this program, you eliminate dairy, gluten, and sugar, as well as caffeine and other foods that are commonly inflammatory.

But at the same time they have a whole list of fruits and vegetables that you can eat, and brown rice (the little bit of starch you're allowed to have). Standard Process also adds good nutrients, green food supplements, herbs that detox the liver, and fiber that attaches to the toxins that are being released from the liver!

People should definitely listen to their bodies . . . if their bodies are healthy. But if you've been abusing your body for years, it's not communicating effectively anymore. After years of eating unhealthy foods, your body has been desensitized. Your gut tried to communicate at some point, but you just beat it down.

At that point you have to go back to, "What do we know is right and true?" That is why I love that purification program. It clears out almost everything and starts you back eating the right way.

It takes twenty-one days to start any new habit, so their three-week diet helps you develop the lifestyle change of eating salads and similar real foods that your body is designed to eat. So you're feeding your body what it needs while it's getting rid of the junk at the same time.

Also, it gives the body time to go through the rejuvenation process, to avoid putting stress on the liver spontaneously. It gives your body time to do what it needs to do.

I also love the purification program because you can eat through it. No feeling deprived of food.

There are a lot of detox diets out there that I don't condone. Those programs are generally shorter, and they're more like fasting. They only give you lemon water, juices, and the like. Unfortunately, our society is so sickly, our bodies are so polluted, that fasting is almost dangerous because our bodies don't have enough nutrients to support them through a fasting process. Fasting can also irritate the organs, because they're not prepared for it.

I've had patients call because they went on one of these poor detox diets and have had serious side effects or go into pancreatitis after starting on a fasting detox diet, because fasting is spontaneous, and their bodies go, "What? You polluted me and now you all of a sudden want me to get rid of this stuff and not feed me?"

Like I said, it takes about a week for a papercut to heal, but it's going to take a lot longer for your gut to heal. Most people notice a difference well within twenty-one days.

The Standard Process diet also helps people who are diabetic or pre-diabetic to detox their livers. Many people who have been pre-diabetic have gotten their sugars under control.

Here's another great advantage: A majority of people lose weight on the purification diet.

Right now we have a lot of "beach body" or 90 day programs, commercials being thrown at us on late-night TV. It's just funny. I crack up, because if anybody commits to a cleaner, healthier diet and lifestyle, and commits to doing any physical activity regularly, they're going to see a positive change. And if they stick with it for three months, they're going to see significant change in their bodies. It's the commitment not the program.

As another option, you could do a food elimination diet using the book *The Elimination Diet: Discover the Foods That Are Making You Sick and Tired—and Feel Better Fast* by Tom Malterre and Alissa Segersten. Countless people have had excellent results from the book and diet.

As your body heals on your elimination diet, your food cravings will dissipate and your stomach will tell you when it's comfortably full. You'll eat less.

I discovered that I have an oat sensitivity and a grain sensitivity. As a kid I'd eat oatmeal. Everyone told me this is what healthy food was, that oats are healthy. Even in the commercials, oats are good. But it always gave me a stomach ache.

I should have realized oats are not good for *me*! My body is different.

So is yours. You need to listen to it. Ask yourself: "Wait a second, what is my body truly saying?"

Go on an elimination diet, and evaluate how your body responds to each food. Listen to the symptoms. What are the symptoms truly telling you?

I grew up eating oatmeal, and it gave me bellyache, but I was told it was healthy. "That's what healthy should feel like, then," I thought.

In college I ate a granola bar and had the same reaction. That's when I started opening my mind to: "Wow, my body's saying it doesn't like this."

Now looking back, I realize I had a grain sensitivity for a long time. Society keeps saying, "But it's healthy!" I've made my own conclusion after really sitting down and thinking about it. "If I eat this, it will not be a good thing, it will not have positive symptoms, for me."

Just because it's good for everyone else doesn't mean it's good for you. You have to find what's good for *you*.

That's what an elimination diet does. It gives you the nutrients, and removes inflammatory offenders, that enable your body to begin really healing.

Additional Benefits of an Elimination Diet

Here is another benefit of an elimination diet. After a few weeks detoxing on the diet, many people suddenly notice that the organic foods they're eating taste more flavorful and more *clean*, especially grass-fed meat. (And that's without artificial flavor enhancers!) After the diet they don't want to go back to non-organic, especially non-organic meats, because those meats no longer taste clean.

Also, since your elimination diet reintroduces what is a normal-healthy functioning body, you may be surprised what you discover about your healthier digestive system afterward.

I have one patient who knows the value in paying attention to what she eats, because she discovered through an elimination diet that red food dye gives her migraines. That non-food caused major side effects. Her immune system said, "I don't like it. It's not food, it's not right, and it irritates me. Get it away from me!" So she eliminated red food dye, along with anything that had red food dye. If she gets a headache now, she asks herself, "Oh, what did I eat?" And she can usually find the source that was the smoking gun.

After the elimination diet, you may notice your body reacting if you try processed food. It might go, "Whoa, hey, red flag! This junk food isn't good for you. I don't like this!" Then you think, "Wow! I didn't realize that caused me to have indigestion." Or a headache.

My son knows. He didn't grow up eating gum. Now that he's in high school, if he tries a piece of gum, with artificial sweeter, his body reacts. "That stuff makes me sick, Mom!"

Other Diet Programs—Worth Checking Out?

Diet programs. I cringe at diet programs where you have to eat their food that isn't healthy food. During their television commercials with smiling celebrity endorsements, the TV camera pans over pizzas and cheeseburgers and all kinds of heavily processed foods, and it's their food, and it helped her lose fifty pounds (which she keeps gaining back).

I see those commercials and think, "You're still eating bread! Bread is one of the big offenders, and that's one of the reasons you've been battling weight gain for the last thirty years!"

Get rid of the bread!

Also, you're still eating other foods that continually cause inflammation. You're not allowing your digestive tract and gut lining to heal. And until that heals, the inflammation will continue. The symptoms will continue. Our bodies' primary need isn't fewer calories. Our bodies' primary need is the nutrients that will allow them to heal.

Many are using commercialized diets and programs. Don't get me wrong, a few are pretty good at trying to teach you discipline. Others aren't. Just buying their food isn't good because that's not teaching you anything. They're feeding you and portioning it for you, so you're dependent on them. You pay them to feed you. So you can lose some weight, but as soon as you stop their program, if you still haven't learned how to portion your meal sizes and make healthy choices, you'll gain back the weight.

You should know your serving sizes, and your portion sizes. So go on the Internet, pull up "serving size chart," and you'll know it's half a cup of this, two-thirds a cup of that. A large banana is technically two serving sizes. A deck of cards is how big your steak or fish should be. It shouldn't cover half your plate. That's too much meat. (That's another reason why the digestive system gets stressed; it struggles to digest so much extra food)

At least half your plate should be fruits and vegetables. Again, an elimination diet will reveal which foods your body needs and which foods it reacts to.

Learning serving sizes can be a good way to start eating healthier quantities.

Several years ago a study came out to evaluate how many people eat according to the government's food pyramid—not a good model, but it's the model everyone learns about in school. The study showed that only about 5 percent eat according to the pyramid. In other words, 95 percent of the population doesn't eat what they think is supposed to be healthy anyway.

A Good Long-Term Diet

I actually don't favor any one, specific long-term diet. I tell my patients, "If you have a diet that's worked very well for you, you function well on it, you feel good on it, you don't have any symptoms coming out, and your bloodwork looks good, then that's great. Do it."

If they love the diet, and it works well for them, great!

I still tell them that my biggest focus is that they get rid of the big offenders. These are the three big ones that are inflammatory:

- ✗ dairy

    ✗   gluten

    ✗   sugar

Again, I tell patients to give those up for at least two to three weeks. And people with strong sensitivities to them should give them up for two to three months before trying them again.

Eat "back to nature," the cleanest foods possible—less hormones, less added ingredients, less all those unnatural things.

Go with fruits, vegetables, and healthy proteins. Just keep it down to that. If you want to use frozen, try to get the flash frozen so that some of the nutrients are intact.

If you have to have a starch, maybe some brown rice. White rice has been processed and bleached. You want to get your rice closest to the natural state as possible.

If you get dry beans, that's okay.

Fish. It seems nobody eats fish anymore, so we're not getting some of the best healthy oils. Our phospholipid layer needs those healthy oils and proteins. So try non-polluted, cold-water ocean fish, such as wild-caught salmon, at least once a week.

Liver—it's a rich source of iron, zinc, and more. We don't eat organ meats like our grandparents did. I remember eating chicken livers, and even a cow liver as a kid—my grandmother was the one who put that in front of me. But my children have no clue what liver tastes like! As a culture we now eat the chicken breasts and legs, and we don't eat those organ meats that have the dense nutrients and minerals that we need. We're vitamin and mineral deficient, some of us severely.

Add liver or organ meats to your diet twice a month. Try to work up to once a week if you want to naturally increase your nutrients in your diet.

Supplements—Be Smart and Beware

Even if you're trying to eat healthy, our plants today are deficient in nutrients since they're over-cropped. And even if you get organic, who's eating five to seven fruits and vegetables a day? Nobody. So you should have a *whole-food based* multivitamin to fill in for the nutrients you're not getting.

Even the allopathic world is recommending multivitamins. Even they admit we're not getting enough nutrients in our foods. The only problem with that is, they're not educated on what over the counter vitamins are.

That takes us to the consumerism of our society. Though manufacturers might sell "A through zinc" multivitamin, a majority of those brands are fragmented vitamins. They're partial vitamins. They're chemically made or chemically distilled.

For example, you can take corn syrup, manipulate it in a lab, and create ascorbic acid. Then you can put ascorbic acid in a pill form, throw it on a shelf, and say, "Okay! That's vitamin C." Because the FDA states, "That's what vitamin C is."

When you evaluate a *real* vitamin C, ascorbic acid is just a shell of what vitamin C is. It's just the outer component. It's not the bioflavonoids or vital nutrients or vital vitamin. It's not the same as eating bell peppers, dark leafy greens, kiwis, an orange, or a pineapple, which are rich in vitamin C. It's not the same as eating buckwheat (it's actually a fruit seed, not a cereal grain), which is highly rich in vitamin C cofactors.

So, you want to make sure you get a *whole-food* supplement, because then you're getting the entire spectrum of nutrients. You're not just getting the fragmented vitamins.

Synthetic, fragmented vitamins can help somewhat, but think about it. If you're trying to turn a key in a lock, and you have a key that only has a couple of ridges, it might work sometimes. It probably won't work well and certainly won't work all the time. Eventually you're going to wear down the key. When we take these fragmented vitamins long-term, that's hard on the system.

"Whole food" is how the bottle should be labeled or described when researched. Read the ingredients on the label. It should say "beet root," "carrot root," "whole food fiber," or "liver." A whole-food label will have ingredients you recognize. You've seen a beet. You've seen a carrot. You know what fiber is. If on the other hand you see ingredients, such as ascorbic acid, and don't know what on Earth it is, then you shouldn't be putting it into your body.

Supplements: Food, Condensed

There's a fear out there caused by all the medical drugs, doses, and side effects. I was on the phone with a woman the other day, advising her to take some supplements, but she was scared to take them. I asked, "Why are you scared of taking the supplements?"

She said, "What if it's too much? I don't want to overdose on it."

I explained, "All I'm giving you is food. Concentrated food. All it'll do is enhance your healing and repair processes. Your body knows how to handle food, and if it doesn't need all of the nutrients, then it'll get rid of the excess. It'll just keep what it needs to heal and discard other parts properly. Are you worried about eating too many salads?"

"No."

I said, "It's the same concept. Your body is going to heal whether you take the supplement or not. The supplement is just going to make it heal faster. So it's up to you. You can take it or not."

She was scared because we've been conditioned to not trust our bodies. So we don't believe our bodies can heal without pharmaceutical drugs.

If you think about it, you will see all the miraculous things our bodies do, like healing papercuts and regenerating our original fingerprints. Our bodies do that, and digest our food, and do thousands of amazing things. But we don't trust our bodies to be able to reverse a cold, or get over an ear infection, or heal from other common illnesses.

Trust your body. With the right nutrients, and the proper communication of the bodies systems, via the nervous system, it can do more than you imagine.

Supplements: The Basic Three

In my office, I provide supplements for patients who need them. The basic, foundational nutritional advise. What I tell people take is:

- a basic whole-food multivitamin (made from actual fruits, vegetables, and plants) and meats
- healthy Omega oil—flax seed oil or fish oil
- a whole food trace mineral complex
- probiotics or eat probiotic rich foods

I advise people to make sure each supplement is a good quality brand usually from a health food store or health professional.

Cheap over the counter supplements are cheap for a reason. Manufactures of supplements that you pick up at the grocery store use inferior or synthesized ingredients because they're in business to make money.

But, you might be thinking, *health food store supplements cost more!* Yes, they do! The reason is that they are made from actual high-nutrient fruits, vegetables, plants, and other sources found in nature, *and* that the holistic science that goes into each supplement does so with the goal of helping your body to actually heal.

So you may think that's a handful of supplements to take a day.

People say, "Ugh, this is too many things to swallow."

I tell them, "I take thirteen supplements on average per day. Thirteen just to stay healthy, because I want to be vital and vibrant when I'm ninety." I want to still be practicing in the office. I want to still be doing what I love. I want to still be helping people.

I'm taking care of my body now because I want to make it to ninety and not be in a nursing home. I'm making that decision now, for my future. I'm investing in myself.

Your health is an investment. You can't afford not to invest in it.

Supplements: How Else Can They Help? (Case Study)

When patients come into my office, they come in primarily for chiropractic. But while they're on the table, I'll ask, "What's going on with your diet? What's going on with your water intake? What's going on with your exercise?" I try to hit those things because I see the difference with the body's improvement.

I want to see people evolve, and get better, and stay healthy, and not just ride the roller coaster of pharmaceutical medications.

For Example, a diabetic patient told me his sugar levels have been high. His medical doctor kept increasing the medicine, but it wasn't making a difference. So I said, "Well there are some things we can talk about nutritionally. Chromium is very important for insulin to be utilized properly. It helps make insulin receptors more sensitive to the insulin.

"So, let's put you on a whole-food supplement that contains higher levels of chromium. See if that will help the insulin to work properly. Maybe you're just lacking the chromium and that's the reason your sugar levels are high."

Cinnamon contains chromium, and this patient was doing the cinnamon, but I suspected he needed even higher levels of chromium. The body will work better with the proper nutrients. Usually when the patient does a diet evaluation, I find out the patients is eating a lot of sugary and refined foods. I advise them to eliminate those bad foods to help decrease the stress on the pancreas.

Beware of Recommendations without Reason

It's not uncommon for the medical world to blanketly say, "Everyone in this category should take this."

Some major medical organizations, for example, state to women over forty, "Every woman over forty should take 500 milligrams of calcium daily."

Their recommended calcium dosage is off the freaking chart, it's so high, and all the while, millions of patients get enough calcium in their diets and their bodies metabolize calcium just fine.

Yet, medical doctors often say, "Everybody should be on this." That's not right!

Even worse (in the instance of calcium) is there are different types of calcium, and most of the calcium on the market is the harshest form of calcium. It's inorganic calcium, calcium carbonate, that's on the shelves. It takes the body approximately thirty-six chemical processes just to get that to be usable, so that's going to be harsher on the body. And we wonder why there is kidney stones or our arthritis is acting up. It's because the body's got all this extra calcium, and it thinks, "I've got to put all this somewhere. Oh, let's shove it into these joints that are irritated, or let's put it wherever."

Most manufacturers don't even reveal what kind of calcium is in the bottle.

However, those that sell their products to health food stores usually will.

A Word of Caution about Vaccines

I'd like to expand on a point here. When it comes to shots, vaccines, or anything you put into your body, the main thing I want you to do is *know what you're putting into your body*. Be mindful of what you're doing.

Ask yourself, "Is this healthy for me?"

Don't just accept, "The doctor says I should do XYZ." My mindful patients challenge me in my own practice, and I am refreshed by that! If I can't explain why I recommend this to you, then I should not be recommending this to you.

If you challenge me on it, sometimes it is frustrating because my initial thought is, "You don't trust my knowledge." But then I think, "I'm happy because that's telling me you're thinking about this, and you're taking ownership on what you want to do to your body."

And I applaud that! I want you to take **ownership** of your body and doing what is healthy for it.

So when one of my patients asks me, "*Why* should I do this?"

If they give me a logical reason why they shouldn't start a treatment I recommended, because of something I missed during the evaluation or wasn't given information about, then I'll say, "Oh, in that case, you're right. We shouldn't do ABC." I'll maybe recommend something else, see what has worked for you in the past, dig up a little more of that history.

So any time you get a blanketed recommendation, you have to sit and consider it. "Well, is that good for me? Is that right for me? Is it right for my child?" Vaccination or not?

Before you decide, you should know what they're putting into you and your child. They should have a list of ingredients that is in whatever they're giving you. You should be able to research to see if it is safe and effective. There are many creditable websites where you can go to research these things. It's your body and your health! It's not enough that someone in a white lab coat says, "Well, we recommend it, because so-and-so told us we need to recommend it, and because so-and-so says this is good."

During decades of manufactures' studies of their own vaccinations, virtually no manufacturer has ever included a true placebo shot. Any shot they compare in studies contains aluminum. Such tests and results are influenced right from the start. They're comparing aluminum to their vaccines.

Be mindful of anything that you put into your body, whether it's anything injected, eaten, or put onto your skin. You need to think, "Is this helping my body, or could it be actually hurting my body?" Then do the research to find out.

We are OWNERS of our bodies! Advocate for yourself! Ask questions! Do your own research before agreeing to anything! Don't blindly accept any "everybody does this" dictate unless there is good reason.

The one thing everyone should be doing is feeding their body the nutrients it needs to heal its self and return to vibrant health.

That's a recommendation *with* reason!

℞ Take OWNERShip—Nutrition

If you want to take this step toward more vibrant health . . .

✓ Switch from nonorganic to organic produce as much as you can to begin healing your body. Organic is best not only because it has fewer additives and fewer pesticides, but it's also much higher in nutrient content.

✓ Try the Standard Process 21-Day Purification Program to purify and support the liver in the detoxification process, this will help discover any food sensitivities you may have.

✓ As another option, you could do a food elimination diet using the book *The Elimination Diet: Discover the Foods That Are Making You Sick and Tired—and Feel Better Fast* by Tom Malterre and Alissa Segersten.

✓ To reduce pain and inflammation, try to avoid the big three inflammatory foods: dairy, gluten, and sugar.

✓ Try eating fish and liver twice a month. Gradually increase until you're having them weekly.

✓ Visit a good health food store and supplement your nutrition with:

  ℞ a basic *whole-food* multivitamin (made from actual fruits, vegetables, and plants)
  ℞ healthy Omega oil—flax seed oil or fish oil
  ℞ a whole food trace mineral complex
  ℞ a good probiotic supplement or food

Exercise Your Passion!

Being OWNERS of our bodies means we should also own what we do with them. The E stands for exercise.

Everybody knows we should exercise, just like everybody knows we should drink eight glasses of water and eat lots of fruits and vegetables.

But *why* exercise? Why not be stagnant?

Because the body was built to move. If you don't exercise, you don't stimulate your blood or circulate your chemistry. You don't nourish your joints. You won't build muscles, which increases natural steroids. Natural steroids help you feel physically, mentally, and emotionally stronger. Then everyday things in life don't seem so tough to deal with. You'll experience more vitality. You'll feel more motivated.

Obviously, exercise stimulates the cells to burn fat. And if you're diabetic, when you exercise you don't need much insulin. Exercise takes stress off the cells to pull in sugars. That takes stress off the pancreas.

Eighty percent of anxiety and depression can be reversed with a consistent exercise program, which helps to release natural endorphins, serotonin, and pain relievers in the brain. (Though nutrients need to be in your body in order to help build those good brain chemicals!)

Exercise also helps push toxins out, and it has a lot of other benefits.

How to Stick with It

With exercise, it all comes back to the commitment of following through. In our society, we are good starters, but poor finishers! Yes, we can get excited about a concept, but do we really have to wait until we're diabetic or have a heart attack to make a change? Really?

So how do you follow through?

1. Do What You Love

Just find something that works for *you*. I'd be the last person to tell you to do any exercise that you don't have a passion for.

Find—and exercise—your passion.

One of my patients, an older lady, had a basement and wanted to roller-skate. People said to her, "What? Are you nuts?"

I told her, "That's Great! You're getting active. Just be safe"

Put some bumpers on the walls if you need to. People were worried about her breaking a hip bone, but actually, if she uses that hip, it gets stronger. If she wants to roller skate, let her roller skate! I applaud her!

Another patient likes to line dance. Find what makes you happy.

For me, if I want to run, I need music. I need good, inspiring, pumping music to help me keep going. If I had to run to silence, I couldn't do it. So I've got to have something help me stimulate my mind, to help me do my running. If I walk, I read while I walk on the treadmill.

2. Start Easy

Another effective way to follow through is to start easy.

You'll be jazzed to hear that exercise—doesn't need to take a lot. As always, keep it simple. You just need to get your body moving.

If you're not active, start off with just five minutes, three times a week. Just be consistent.

If there is a physical activity you have a passion for, do that. If there is no physical activity you enjoy, just do a little walking.

To people who don't exercise, starting off with half an hour a day, five days a week, is way too much—of course people quit. It takes three weeks to establish a new habit. So only do five minutes, three times a week.

What you might find is that knowing you can stop in five minutes feels so freeing (and energizing!) that you'll actually walk a little longer. If so, great! If you only walk five minutes, great! Put it on your calendar for the next three weeks to walk five minutes, three times a week. Then you'll have established a habit.

After three weeks, add another five minutes per day. Or add another day per week. *Gradually* increase what you can do, until you're walking ten minutes a day, four or five days per week. Do that for at least another three weeks, until you've established that habit.

Then try to do fifteen minutes a day, five days a week.

By letting yourself slowly get into the groove of a healthy new habit, you'll be far more likely to stick with it and benefit from it.

If you have a physical condition where you can't walk, go on YouTube and find videos that lead you in stretching or simple yoga. Find something that gets you stretching and creating some kind of activity to move those muscles. Follow those videos until you feel like you can do some walking or another activity that gives you good all-over body conditioning and blood circulation.

Optimally, how much exercise should everyone be getting? Thirty to forty-five minutes, five times a week.

The best thing you can do is just get started. Five minutes a day, three days a week. That alone helps most people to start feeling more energetic.

3. Be Encouraged

Find what works for you and what inspires you to follow through. Don't give up because you can only make it ten days. If you made it ten days, excellent! Good try! Get back on the horse, and let's start again.

Trying it that way didn't work? So, let's try it *this* way. There are hundreds of ways we can do things. We don't have to do it a certain way.

Nowadays, you can go to any gym and take classes. You can watch fitness videos. You can stream exercise videos online. You have an endless variety out there, so don't give up if you failed the first time, second time, or third time. Just keep going until you find what works for you.

And once you find what works for you, then you feel great! It's amazing.

Find encouraging people in your life. Find those support groups. Me personally—I used to go to a twenty-four-hour fitness place. After three months you've established relationships with the people who always come at the same time. It's funny how we form a casual group. If I didn't come for a week, they'd say, "Where were you last week? What's going on?"

"I was on vacation," or, "I was at a conference." There's an inner accountability when you find like-minded people and have that support system.

So, once you find your activity, find a community of like-minded people who like the same thing you do. And that will help you perpetuate your activity as well.

If you outgrow them? Move on to the next group. It's okay! It's okay to move beyond people who don't grow with your mind-set. Surround yourself with people you admire, people who are doing the things you want to do. That's going to help a lot. Find that support system.

Some people are motivated by big events like maybe running in a 5K or looking good for a wedding. A good way to get some leverage on yourself is to have a reason or goal to exercise.

Do what you love, start easy, and be encouraged. That'll inspire you to exercise your passion . . . and to follow through!

ꙮ Take OWNERShip—Exercise

If you want to take this step toward more vibrant health . . .

- ✓ Write on your calendar to exercise five minutes, three times a week, for the next three weeks, doing something you *enjoy*. Then you'll have established a habit.
- ✓ After three weeks, add another five minutes per day. Or add another day per week.
- ✓ *Gradually* increase what you can do, until you're exercising your passion ten minutes a day, four or five days per week. Do that for at least another three weeks, until you've established that habit.
- ✓ Then try to do fifteen minutes a day, five days a week.
- ✓ Try to gradually work toward exercising thirty to forty-five minutes, five times a week.
- ✓ Find encouraging people to exercise with that will help hold you accountable.

Rest to Renew You

Up till now we've taken OWNERShip of our oxygen, water, nutrition, and exercise. The primary benefit of those is to heal the body. But a secondary benefit is to heal the mind.

By focusing now on the R, rest, we're going to switch that around. We're going to focus on restoring vibrant health to the mind, though you will see the body will also benefit.

As I said earlier, in our fast-paced, blitz-through-life society, almost no one gets enough rest. We pack kids' schedules tight with school and year-round extracurricular activities. We pack our own schedules with so much work we wish we could be cloned. We even pack our weekends and vacations with activities.

As a culture and as individuals, we desperately need to become OWNERS of our rest. Our minds can't be refreshed and our bodies can't heal well if we don't take sufficient time to recover.

Go to Bed!

First of all, we are not sleeping enough hours. We should be getting eight hours a night of *restful* sleep, on average. But everyone's body is different. If someone's body really needs nine hours, then they should not limit themselves to eight hours!

However, research has shown if you sleep more than ten hours, it's counterproductive. That's because you're releasing more cortisol, an adrenal hormone that can lead to physical irritation with too much amounts of sleep and that's more damaging. You know you've slept too much if you get up and you're stiff and uncomfortable. When you get up, you should feel refreshed. You should feel like you have energy for the day.

Obviously, if you feel like you're sick, you probably need more rest or sleep than usual.

Find what works optimally for you, what you feel like you need.

What's Your Sleep Style?

How should you sleep? Traditionally everyone should be sleeping on their backs, with the neck adequately supported on a pillow four to five inches deep, which research has shown. I generally recommend a pillow underneath the knees to help relax the lower back.

If you like to sleep on your side, make sure you have support and healthy alignment—your shoulder, hip, and knees in a straight line, with a pillow between the knees so the hips aren't rotating forward or backward. Try to stack the knees so everything is symmetrical, with the body in a neutral spinal position.

Rhythm and Blues

What is the optimal sleeping rhythm? The more sleep you get in the evening, the best it is. So if you don't go to bed until midnight, that's typically not as restful. So if you work nights, that definitely throws off the body's rhythm. The best timing for deep sleep is between nine at night and seven in the morning.

Do what you can. Try to get a good eight hours in.

If you occasionally share sleep space with pets or small children, your subconscious mind is going to be worrying, monitoring them, and you won't sleep as well. Particularly the moms. Some little movement or cry or whimper, and you're like, "Okay, what's going on?" Obviously this may be good for bonding, but most times children and pets should have their own sleeping areas with their space to move. There's a point where children need to have their own independence and their own beds to learn how to sleep in restful positions and develop good sleeping habits.

Dogs and cats pester you, wake you up, and take over the bed. They don't really care how well you sleep. *They* want to be comfortable.

Some people may need the protection of a dog or the closeness of a pet. They need something that helps them feel more secure. And that makes them able to sleep better. If that is the case, be sure to weigh whether or not you actually sleep better and feel more refreshed in the morning.

Take Vacations.

The other aspect of rest—or more accurately, lack of rest—in our society is that people don't take vacations. We don't take time. Or maybe we do take vacations, but the planning and getting to destinations becomes so stressful that by the time we're on vacation, we can't really enjoy it. We're too stressed out trying to decompress from traveling.

And while on vacation, we're worried about the jobs we're coming back to, because we know there's going to be a pile on the desk.

I say take a quarterly vacation—time just to unplug from work and stress, time to reset and to enjoy self-reflection and life. Be sure to take that time. It doesn't have to be a long week. But I do recommend taking at least two weeks a year—one week at a time, or both weeks at once—where you are totally free of anything to do.

Try a Stay-cation!

Also take long, three- or four-day weekends whenever you feel stress beginning to build so you don't let yourself reach a point of ongoing inner tension.

You can do multi-day stay-cations too, where you say, "I'm just going to hang out at home and not do anything," or plan fun things locally that you enjoy.

The goal with long weekends and stay-cations is to not do anything that you're consistently always doing. Unplug and mix it up. New experiences are really important to renew your mind and spirit.

The more stressful your job, the more you need to escape the normal and get refreshed.

Take time with your family. Enjoy nature. Take time to be creative.

I love my job, but for my recent stay-cation, I did something new and picked up one of those creative coloring books. Coloring, I discovered, taps parts of my brain that I don't use that often. And it was so great because when I came back to the office, I was ready to come back. I was excited to come back. And I arrived with a new perspective. I had a couple of complicated cases, and the stay-cation brought about fresh ideas that I hadn't thought of before.

Those fresh perspectives are needed.

Rest Every Weekend

We need to rest on regular weekends too. We need to have one day every week completely free. Nobody rests on the weekends anymore. Everybody's running around, catching up, doing the grocery shopping, doing this, doing that. Taxes the kids. Etc....

Nobody truly sits and really just hangs out at home with no agenda. But we need to, every weekend. Or we need to set times aside during the week where we say "I'm not going to do anything. We're going to just rest." That is so freeing!

Always being on the go is cultural. It's our society. Society wants to strap us to a fast-moving train that never stops. People in other countries around the world know when to stop and rest. In areas of the US such as the Bible Belt, people stop and rest. They go to church on Sunday, but afterward, they have lunch and just hang out. No agenda. No plans.

When you take enough time to rest, or be creative and do something interestedly inspiring then your worktime is more productive.

A Rest-less Culture

When people work two, three jobs, and don't take time to unplug and rest, the next thing you know, they have cancer. They have leukemia. You can't run your body like that. The body needs rest. The mind needs rest.

I frequently get emergency calls from patients I've never seen before. "I'm leaving on vacation tomorrow, and I just threw my back out." It's very interesting. They push and push their bodies, telling themselves, "I'm going to be on vacation soon." But their bodies decide, "You're going to rest *now*. I'll make sure you rest; I'm throwing you off. Enough!"

Here's another problem. As a society, we're in such a hurry to do so much, even while on vacation. When people take vacations today, the trips go something like this: "We went on this cruise, and there were opportunities for us to run here and run there and do this and do that excursion, and we did it all."

My family and I did that, one time. We signed up for excursions at every port. Then they ran us here and ran us there, all throughout every day, and we had to be back on the boat by eight o'clock every night. I felt more stressed when I came back because of the agendas I'd had to follow.

The next cruise we went on, my husband, kids, and I were more relaxed. Other family members who came along kept pressuring us, saying, "Did you sign up for the excursion? Did you do—?"

I said, "Nope. I don't know what we'll do then. I have a list of options. We'll think about it tomorrow morning when we get up and see what we want to do."

Your vacation should not feel stressed. So don't take a vacation with a relative that drives you nuts, the relative that adds stress to you, whether that be your mom, sister, or someone else. Vacations are for rest. Plan separate family time some other time if you need to.

Take ownership. Be mindful. Ask yourself, "Is this restful? Do I actually enjoy this?"

What is restful and joyful for you is not necessarily good for someone else. Do what's best for *you*. Find those things.

Rest to heal your body, and to restore vibrant health to your mind.

ॐ Take OWNERShip—Rest

If you want to take this step toward more vibrant health . . .

✓ Try to get eight hours of deep, uninterrupted sleep, or however much helps you truly rest each night.
✓ Take a quarterly vacation—time to unplug from work and stress, time to reset and to enjoy self-reflection and life.
✓ Also take long, three- or four-day weekends whenever you feel stress beginning to build so you don't let yourself reach a point of ongoing inner tension.
✓ Rest one day every week. On that day, relax. Do nothing stressful. You need it.

Social Health Externally That Rejuvenates You Internally

Health is physical, mental, social, and spiritual well-being, not just the absence of disease or sickness.

The S that we all need to take OWNERShip of is social health, and mental health is part of it, just as it was part of R—rest.

Our social health is in crisis, in large part due to our culture of stress. When I talk with my patients who are in their nineties, they say, "The stresses that my grandchildren have on them are totally different than the stresses I had. There are more demands on everyone now. And when I grew up, people took time to relax in the evenings." Back then on Sundays, society said that all businesses had to be closed. People knew rest was that important.

Even in my generation—(people now 30s to 40s)—growing up we only had a certain sport at a certain time of the year. We had baseball season, and we had basketball season, and we had volleyball season. Other than three times a year, we didn't have that much going on.

That's no longer how we treat ourselves. Now we have pee wee football and baseball all week, and families are running around all weekend long.

I have full spectrum patients, from elderly to babies, and a lot of families. Every time I ask questions about what activities these little ones are doing, the parents have their children in ballet, in tumbling, and the children have just barely started walking. Many parents of three-year-olds are pressured to have their children in dance or tumbling.

Gymnastics gyms have been popping up. They start teaching very young children whose bodies aren't ready. Yes, small children are okay to play, and I want them to be active. But free playtime has been fading away. Now it's structured play—let's do this dance class, or let's do this.

If you don't have your child in some kind of activity, you're looked at as strange or as if something isn't right. You're weird in our society today. You're almost not seen as a good parent. "Your child should be doing something."

I see kids who are playing baseball all year round. There are kids doing volleyball all year round. That's showing up in the emergency and orthopedic realms. Now, we're getting kids as young as eight years old with repetitive shoulder, elbow, wrist, and knee injuries, because they don't have that season of rest.

Parents aren't guiding their kids to be more free and more energetic. Then when kids come home, they're busy on their tablets and their laptops!

The parents don't understand that we all need to rest—a *lot* more rest than we're getting. If you actually want your kids to perform in high school and college, you can't be doing this to them now. Even Olympic athletes take time off to rest their bodies.

Pressure. Pressure on parents. Pressure on very small children. Even now there's pressure on teenagers before college. In addition to their school load, they have to do extracurricular activities to make sure that they can get into a good school. Add to that the pressure of trying to get scholarships, grants, and other means of financing they can get, because colleges are so expensive and costs are continuing to climb.

Then countless young adults are graduating college with heavy student loan debts, yet are having trouble getting jobs. That's financial stress—yet another serious stress.

Many adults today are under heavy workloads at their offices, and they've got long commutes besides. Several of my patients are spending two hours a day commuting. That's two hours of their lives every day that they can't devote to rest or home.

Almost every single job description today says "exciting, fast-paced environment." That's code for "we're going to pile as much stress on you as we can possibly get away with." It means, "You're going to be stressed working here."

All that stress comes from the pressure of society. Doing what everyone else is doing, being better than anybody else, or comparing yourself to everyone else.

We're getting pushed around by cultural standards. Whether that be the cars we drive, the homes we live in, or whether that be, "Should we decorate for the holidays? Nobody's got their Christmas lights up," repeating what others in the neighborhood do.

It's the social standing of how much money we should be making and how many activities we should be doing.

And it's killing us.

It Really Is Okay—and Healthy!—to Say No

Our society is a culture in crisis. We don't have to accept the stress society would put on us.

Instead, sit down and say, "No. What is best for me and my health? And what is best for my family and my family's health?"

If a mom comes into my office, confides that she feels pressured by other parents to get her daughter involved in more activities, and asks my advice, I say, "First off, let's talk about you. You're overloaded. Let's talk about what you're involved in. What have you overcommitted to?"

The mom will say something like, "You know, I'm in the church choir, and I'm in the mom's group, and I'm in this, and I'm in that."

So I explain, "There are a lot of good things you can be involved in, but you don't have to be in all of them. It's okay to say no."

I actually do a lot of counseling on how to say no. "I test them by stating, I'm going to ask you to do stuff, and you are going to tell me *no*." You might laugh, but I'm not joking. I actually help some of my patients by doing this. I ask them to do something silly and have them practice saying "no" to me.

I'll tell you the same—It's okay to say "no".

How do you know what to say no to? That decision should be based on your values. Do you value that activity? Do you actually, really like it? If you don't value it, if you don't like it, it's okay to say no.

Figure out which activities inspire you and are your passion. For instance, if there was a crisis and you could only choose one activity to do, do that. If you must leave a group, you could say, "It's okay if you feel I have disloyalty or a lack of commitment. I'm going to just pause on the group for a while. I have other priorities."

Maybe you will eventually go back to that activity, or maybe not, but if you're loading yourself down, you need to free up that energy and that time for yourself. Don't wait for society's massive bubble of stress to burst. It's okay to take yourself out of that stress.

When I see the need, I actually write my patients scripts. "Go out with friends." I did that and handed it to a stressed mom once. I said, "Hand this to your husband so he knows you need this. You need your non-mom, non-professional time."

She almost cried. "Oh my gosh!"

I added, "With no guilt. God did not create us to feel guilty. You need time for yourself, and it is okay. It's allowed. It's actually needed! So, it's okay to say, 'No, I'm not going to take care of the kids tonight, honey. You've got this. I'm going out.' It's okay."

I definitely don't mean abandon your whole family! That's silly. But these people are just run down, overloaded. It's amazing how simply doing an occasional night out gives them that sigh of relief and that feeling of, "I'm a person again!"

You should feel free to do the same, then try to make it consistent.

You might even inspire others to do the same. You might find yourself inspiring meaningful change.

It's okay not to have your daughter in Girl Scouts *and* dance *and* tumbling. Also, make sure the kids actually want to do the activities that you have them in. Ask, "Do you actually like this activity? Or are you just doing it because you think it'll make Mom and Dad happy?"

I wish I had a child who played piano. I wanted it, badly. My daughter started piano. She played for three months, maybe a little longer. And then she wouldn't practice. I would urge her to, but she would say, "I don't want to."

I would get upset, but then the piano teacher told me, "If it's not for her, it's not her."

I finally said, "You're right." I didn't keep forcing her to play, even though I had paid all that money for the lessons. Piano just wasn't her thing. Sometime later we got her into band, and she found the flute. She fell in love with the flute, and she practiced it on her own all the time. I didn't even have to ask her to practice.

So, I don't have a piano player, and that's okay, because I want her to be her. We can't impose what we want on other people. We have to let them be who they need to be.

If your child does want to participate in one or two activities, then it's okay to say no to other activities. It's okay to even cycle the activities, saying, "You know what? We're only going to do one activity at a time." And that's good for your kids to realize, to say no to one thing or the other, and start teaching them about time management and prioritizing.

It Really Is Okay to Have YOU Time!

Couples need a date night. They also need that time for themselves. They need a date night with themselves, or their friends, or whatever gives them joy.

Again, first decide what your family's values are and then design activities around them. Find out what's true to your family. You can even find out what's been forced on them, then cut out all the stuff that's not them.

Also, each member of the family, including you, must take time for him- or herself! Think of it like the oxygen mask on an airplane. First put the mask on yourself, then help someone else with their mask. If you're not surviving and breathing yourself, you are not going to be able to take care of other people.

We all need rest. We all need to do things that bring us joy. And we all need healing exercises, physically and mentally.

A mom came into my office last month. She was stressed, overloaded with work. Her corporation is downsizing, so they're having people do twice as much work. The employees are stuck—they do the work to avoid being among those downsized, but they're stressed by the amount of work. So my patient is trying to do the work of two people, and then she goes home at night, and she has toddlers to take care of, even though her husband is helpful.

I asked her, "So, when are you taking time for yourself?" She admitted that she used to enjoy exercising regularly, but she stopped since she was so busy. I said, "Okay, five minutes for yourself a day, of doing whatever exercise or meditation you like. You need to prioritize that. You can carve out five minutes. Do that for yourself. Make it happen! Just five minutes. Set the timer, and do it."

Generally when people come to me, they just don't feel well or are in pain. Somewhere in them, they know they shouldn't feel this way. It might be ongoing symptoms that they're dealing with, so they're usually ready to get help. They're searching for something that will improve their health.

That is, unless their husband or wife says, "You need to get in there." And those patients are not necessarily ready themselves.

In my practice, patients pay out of pocket. Many people who aren't ready to improve their heath don't usually come to me. Because, when people come to me they are ready to invest in their most precious asset, their Health. When they pay, they are subconsciously saying,

"Yes, I'm ready to make a change. I'm willing to pay for it." And they typically make the changes needed to improve their health.

Some of my patients first went to the Mayo Clinic. Mayo doesn't understand the nervous system aspect of chiropractic—how chiropractic can help remove interference and take tension off the nervous system. Because not only do we chiropractors adjust people's skeletal structure (everybody thinks of chiropractors as relieving pain and headaches), but we're also removing tension on the nerves, and nerves are the master control system for the whole body. So when you remove the tension, it gives the body a higher capacity to deal with things. So we take that pressure off, and that helps the body heal and thrive tremendously.

Taking that time and doing all that for yourself is so important.

But the external stressors that cause internal tension still have to change.

What Changes Can You Make to Destress Your Mind?

1. Declutter It

Mental health. What can you do to have a healthier mind? First, declutter it.

Once a week, try to sit down and unload your brain on a piece of paper. List the things you need to get done. Make plans. Set goals. Then take a few minutes to organize your plans and goals. Once you have, you no longer have that energy burning in the back of your mind. You no longer have to think about it.

It's such a relief to do that! And it's funny, because when you have, all of a sudden things start happening to assist you to get those things accomplished. When you're able to focus on one thing instead of mentally juggling several, things get done faster and better.

So bring those plans and goals to the front and clean them out.

Find other ways to declutter your mind. I heard a story once that while Albert Einstein was being interviewed, the reporter asked if he could have Einstein's phone number so he could call if he had further questions. "Certainly" replied Einstein and went to the phone book and looked up his number, wrote it on a slip of paper and handed it to the reporter. Surprised, the reporter said, "You are considered to be the smartest man in the world and you can't remember you own phone number?"

Einstein replied, "Why should I memorize something when I know where to find it."

Prioritize what you want to put into your brain, what actually needs to be in there and what doesn't.

In my practice, I pull out books all the time and look up things. Years ago when I worked as an assistant for a medical doctor, I remember the medical doctor slipping out of the exam room and running to his office to look up information. Then he'd run back in and act like he'd known it all along. I'm free to say that I'm a real person. I openly tell patients, "You know what, I don't remember the answer exactly, but I know where to look to find it. Let me look that up quick. I want to make sure I'm telling you the right information and giving you the right advice and recommendations so we can get you better."

Declutter. Why? Because our brains are not infinite. But there is infinite information out there that we can easily access.

2. Choose Your Viewpoint

Second, improve your mental health by stepping back and finding your mental stress. Where is it coming from? Is it actually a physical stress because you're not taking care of your body and that is affecting you mentally? Or do you maybe have stress because you're a worrier?

Some people just gravitate to being worriers. Take those thoughts captive and realize you have a choice to change them! I've heard of research revealing that 80 to 90 percent of stuff we worry about will either never happen, or are things we have no control over. So what's the point of worrying about it? Worrying changes nothing. I have heard a worry is a wish for something you don't want.

> Focus on the things you can change,
> let go of the rest,
> and move on.

You have to realize if you're a worrier. If you are, you have to take an active road to change because your thoughts create your reality.

You can also change your worries into gratitude. Have that attitude of gratitude! Change your fear into faith! With some patients who have a tendency to worry, I assign them to do a gratitude exercise: Keep a gratitude journal. Write in it every morning, night, or any time you take a step toward that worry place. Rather than write your worries, write what you're grateful for. Write what is good and going well.

Rather than worry, switch it around. Start thinking, "Okay, what blessings do I have? What things am I grateful for?" You might write, "My family is healthy. I have a nice home. I have a nice car. . . ."

Once you start that new focus, you're switching the whole pathway. That mind-set helps everything. When you continue it to become a habit, then the habit of worrying will disappear.

Also, start each day off right. You have a choice on how you want to start each day. You can say, with dread, "Good God, it's Monday." Or you can say, with excitement and gratitude, "Good God, it's Monday."

Sometimes, I admit, I wake up dreading the day ahead. "Oh, it's going to be a horrible day. I have so much I have to get done!" Then I have to make myself think, "I have a lot on my plate today, but it's going to be great, and everything's going to work out." Then I have to repeat the positive version with an excited tone over and over—three, four, sometimes seven or eight times—before I actually believe it.

That's a *choice*. I choose not to keep my mind in the negative. We have a choice to redirect, to start each day on the right foot. Choose to believe things will go well, and most often they will.

Visualize Your Optimal Life

Visualization is very important, because it helps your mind to actually see what you want. What you actually strive for.

I want my two kids to find their calling, so I take a few minutes now and then and visualize them happy, wearing their graduation caps, ready to start the new phase of their lives. I envision that, and it makes me smile. It makes me happy. It gives me positive energy to help them.

When you visualize what you want to be and achieve, it's amazing how things start to happen. I'll admit, I was a sceptic when I first heard about visualizations, but then I tried them. Now I recommend them to everyone who wants to succeed.

Many sports coaches have their teams visualize themselves making winning plays. They have tremendous results. According to research, visualization is just as important as doing the physical practice themselves.

It dissolves your fear. It gives you power. It results in success.

If a person doesn't have a mental vision of where they're going, or if a corporation doesn't have a clear vision of their mission, they aren't going to thrive. They aren't going to grow. They'll just say, "Whatever, get through the day."

You can visual the optimal future and bring that about. Or you can visualize the negative and bring that about. What you consistently focus on, you become.

Then the key to self-help is to act as-if. Act as if you're already there. Feel as if you're already there. That changes your mind-set and helps you achieve it.

3. Engage in Self-discovery

The third way to have a healthier mind has to do with whether you're a left brain person or a right brain person. The analytical side verses the creative and imaginative. Our society supports more of the analytical—numbers, exactness. They cater to that more than to the artistic.

Yes, they do offer art classes, but that's limited throughout elementary school and high school, as is drama. That lack of creative outlet has a long-term negative effect on the mind health of right brain students.

If you're a right brain person, keep your mind health strong by regularly doing activities such as math problems, studying a new language, or increasing your computer skills. If you're a left brain person, engage often in activities that appeal to your creative side. Sculpt, paint, color. Do things with your hands, even if you're weak at it; just do something fun. Or just sit and look at nature, enjoy its beauty, and feel its presence.

Be purposeful in caring for your mind health. Strengthen the side of your mind that craves an outlet. It's amazing how that will help everything come together and balance out.

It will increase your energy and your clarity of thought.

4. Consider New Possibilities for Your Career

Are you stressed by your job? Some people feel hopeless in their jobs. They feel stuck. If this is speaking to you, then how can you adapt better at work or eliminate the stress from work?

Is your attitude negative when you walk into work? How might you change your attitude? Can you listen to positive music on the way there? Can you listen to your favorite author's novels on CD? Can you listen to CDs of your favorite comedian? Those can give you a joyful ride there, and then you're starting the day much more positively.

Or you can have a healthier mind by working the right job for your right or left brain. For example, if you're a logical left brainer, you may be constantly stressed by working in a loosely structured environment. And if you're highly creative, then it may be stressful, and potentially damaging to your health, for you to stay long-term in a firmly structured or an intensely analytical job.

If you're an introvert, you may be stressed in a highly populated environment. If you're an extrovert, you'll likely be stressed in a setting that has few employees.

If you tend to work a little more slowly than others, an "exciting, fast-paced environment" will pile on the stress. If you tend to work quickly, a job with a limited number of tasks will cause frustration and tension to build.

Stress is a mountainous obstruction to good physical, mental, and emotional health.

If you're forced into a career, position, or working environment that is not well suited for you, that will cause you mental stress. It will constantly tax you. It will dampen your spirit, the thing that drives you underneath. You'll likely become depressed.

Don't get me wrong—you should still strengthen yourself and grow, but if you do too much of what doesn't suit you, for too long, then your mental health will suffer until you correct the situation.

Should you change your job?

The tendency is to be the victim and say, "No-no-no. I can't possibly change my job!" Everybody acts like they don't have an option. People are so skittish of change that they keep living under mountains of stress.

Let's step back and consider, "Okay, what can we change? Let's identify things we can change." Okay, you feel stuck in this job. Have you actually tried to get a different job? If you tell me no, then let's talk about that. Are you truly, truly stuck?

If you change 1 percent of 50 things, then technically you've changed 50 percent of things, right? Those little changes are going to cause a big effect.

So think about one little thing you can change. Then another. And then another.

Take ownership. It's your job to say, "Oh, I can change *these* things." It's your responsibility to say, "Yes, I can take these steps."

If you start looking, really looking, you'll find there's an abundance of possibilities.

Most patients come into my chiropractic office because they have physical manifestations of mental stress. They don't like their jobs and all the related tension. Often the jobs demand more of them than they are able to put out physically and/or mentally. And they really don't like what they're doing, whether it be ethically or the skills they must use.

But they don't feel confident enough to step out of their comfort zones and go find what would best suit them. Fact is, most don't really know what suits them because they haven't tried to find which career fits their personalities, what their purpose is, or where their talents are. So they're stuck in their jobs. They know they're not happy where they work, and that work is nerve-wracking, but they don't know where to go. They just float like helpless driftwood in the current, year after year.

Instead, ask yourself, "Can this be better? How can I change things?"

Discover your personality type, purpose, talents, skills, and your values. Those make up your blueprint. Those are what drive you.

How do you discover them? Search online for "personality test." You'll find several, all with easy questionnaires to answer. Take free tests by Myers-Briggs, Strengths Finder, Enneagram, and DISC. Gain a lot of information about yourself.

When you take those tests, it's funny because you just start laughing, "Yeah, that's me!" Those tests help you really accept yourself, since you realize, "Okay, I am unique, because everybody has a different blend of all these different talents and skills. But, I'm also not unusual. This is simply me. This is how I am. It's okay to be me. A lot of other people have the same little ticks, quirks, and pluses."

One of my mentors used to say, "Each personality style equally sucks and equally is great." Every personality has its pros and cons. Every personality has good parts.

What's great is that when I first started doing the personality research, I saw that I gravitated toward being unhealthy. For example, my personality tends to be indecisive. So I often spent quite a bit of time before going to work just looking at my closet, thinking, "Do I want to wear blue today? Should I do my hair up or down?"

I've learned to think, "Just pick something and go!"

It's cool to say, "Okay, that's the weakness in my personality. So I understand that, and here's how to overcome it."

Once you've gained a lot of information about yourself studied the results. Search "[your personality type], careers." Search "list of values" to discover more about which career and environment are likely to fit you best.

It's critical to be purposeful, mindful, and to figure yourself out.

Unfortunately, many people have barriers to getting into the jobs they really want, barriers such as getting new college degrees. Do whatever is necessary to get yourself free of daily job stress! You'll thrive in a career, position, or working environment that fits your personality and interests.

I've had several patients who've identified their jobs as a huge cause of their stress and then said, "You know what? I'm going to look for a better job that suits me." And they find a better job. And their health improves.

I've had patients who've demoted themselves. They've said, "This is not right. I did better when I was a lower position. I was better as a worker than as management, which they brought me up to. I want to go down, and it's fine if I lose the money."

It's such an amazing thing when those patients come back in and say, "Oh my gosh! Things are so much better now! By so much!"

They recognize that sometimes the money's not worth it. Don't get me wrong—you can find work that better suits you *and* that pays you better.

If you are in the right spot, you're happy. You have freedom. You have energy.

If you get pushed into another position, evaluate. Is this position possibly better for you? Maybe you can find a new way to excel with your talents and skills, with that demotion, or with the other pathway, the other journey. That's something to really look at.

So declutter; start each day with a positive outlook; regularly fulfil the cravings of your left or right brain; and discover the right career, position, and working environment for your personality and interests. That will help you to destress long-term and to thrive with greater mental health.

℞ Take OWNERShip—Social Health

If you want to take this step toward more vibrant health . . .

- ✓ Are you or your children overcommitted? It's okay to say no and to prioritize.
- ✓ Each member of the family, including you, must take time for him- or herself, to rest and to do things that bring you joy.
- ✓ To destress your mind:
    - ℞ Once a week, try to sit down and unload your brain on a piece of paper. List the things you need to get done. Make plans. Set goals. Then take a few minutes to organize your plans and goals.
    - ℞ Keep a gratitude journal. Write in it every morning, night, or any time you take a step toward that worry place. Rather than write your worries, write what you're grateful for. Write what is good and going well.
    - ℞ Visualize what you want to be and achieve. It dissolves your fear. It gives you power. It results in success. What you consistently focus on, you become.
    - ℞ Engage in self-discovery. Exercise your right and left brain. Do activities that in engage both sides of the brain.

> ℞ Should you change your job? Consider it. Allow for the possibility that something better exists. Then discover your personality type, purpose, talents, skills, and your values. You'll thrive in a career, position, or working environment that fits your personality and interests.

What Changes Can You Make to Destress Your Family?

In our society, we basically go with the flow. However, it's our job as parents to be advocates for our children, to find out our children's personality styles, and to factor in those personality styles with their education and activities.

For example, introverts might do well around people, be outgoing or have fun, but they need alone time to recharge. Some children need a lot of that alone time, or they need quiet time with their families. Their parents and families need to let them know that it's okay. You shouldn't necessarily make them alone; you can do things together in a relaxing way.

So discover your children's personality types. Then you can best understand what and how they think, what life is like from their perspectives, how best to (and not to) parent them, and what careers will most likely appeal to them. That will greatly reduce your children's (and your) stress. Then they'll enjoy better mental and physical health, since the two are closely related.

It's also mentally healthy for kids (and parents) to unplug electronic devices and have "No Screen Day." Have a day each week or designated times where no one is plugged into the Internet, computer, phones, TV, or any technology. Just decide, "we're going to play board games, read, color, work some crafts, do a puzzle, or we're going to do something else."

Say you're more of an introverted or withdrawn parent, and you like to be more of a homebody, but your child's more outgoing. Then especially you need, and they need, that parent-child connectedness and belonging. They also need to be involved in groups to meet their outgoing needs.

So monitor your family time and activities. Cater to their personality types. Also, know their (and your) love languages. Read *The 5 Love Languages of Children*, *The 5 Love Languages of Teenagers*, and discover your own and your spouses in *The 5 Love Languages*, all by Gary Chapman.

Knowing personality types, how they interact, and what each needs, makes a phenomenal difference in raising a healthy child and close family.

A lot more teachers are more open to children's personality types nowadays. When my two children were in kindergarten, I discovered a distinct difference between them as far as right brain and left brain. My son is very much like me, very analytical, so in kindergarten when he was learning his letters and writing his name, homework was easy. I'd give him a plain paper and a pencil and say, "Write your name five times."

He'd say, "Okay." Then he'd sit down with the paper and pencil, and he'd write it.

Now then, my daughter went to the same class. I'd say, "Let's sit down and practice writing your name."

She'd write it twice and then say, "I'm bored! I don't want to do this!"

At the time, I wasn't as knowledgeable about right and left brain. So I sighed and went to the teacher. "She won't do the homework!"

The teacher told me, "She's more creative. More tactile. You need to get a dry erase board and different colors of markers. You can do it that way."

She was right, and the best kindergarten teacher I've ever come across.

After that I'd set out the dry erase board and markers. I'd tell my daughter, "Write your name in different colors, but you need to write it at least ten times." Then she could do it. She would do her homework, and do the things that we needed her to do.

I praise God that I got that experience early on and realized, "Okay, she's a creative kid. For homework, we've got to color. We've got to draw."

But my son is like, "I can just read a book."

So find out who your child is. Help them discover themselves. Help them find their calling, their purpose in life, and to fulfill it.

Today my daughter is in drama, and my son is strongly academic.

It's also very important to make sure you don't put emphasis on either side of the right-brain, left-brain discussion. During my son's first semester in high school, he earned a 4.2 GPA. We praised him for it. "That's great."

My daughter is more of a B or C average student. She responded, "I'm dumb. I'm stupid. I'm ___." She started the negative self-talk.

I quickly reminded her, "Don't let anybody talk to you, even yourself, in a negative way. Don't tell yourself you're stupid. Don't tell yourself anything negative. Flip that around and say, 'No, I'm beautiful. I'm amazing. I'm creative. I'm smart. Don't take that away from yourself.'"

I actually pulled out references of Einstein. In elementary school his teachers sent him home from school and said, "We can't teach him. He's too stupid to teach."

His mom told him, "We're just going to homeschool you."

In time he found a good mentor who catered to him, and his extraordinary abilities came to light.

I told my daughter, "Someone like Einstein was told he was stupid, but he wasn't. He just needed to find where he would thrive. So you can't compare yourself to your brother or your friends. You are unique. As long as you're trying your best and doing the things you need to do, I'm not going to let you say, 'Oh I'm not good enough.' You are good in drama, whereas your brother is not. And you're good in other things. So whatever sparks your passion, your interests, those are the things you should go on with. That's what we need to strengthen. That might not show up in grades, but it's going to show up somewhere else. We're not going to measure grades."

It's important for every parent to learn the personality types and the gifts and abilities of their children, and not to impose their own personality type on them.

Parenting Behavior That Influences Children's Health

Often people talk about genetics. But a lot of times we inherit lifestyle and behavior patterns from our parents as well. Because that's how they are, and how they do things, you automatically think that's how things should be done.

I love the story about the granddaughter who is roasting a ham. She cuts the ends off the ham and puts the middle of the ham in the oven to bake it. Her husband asks, "Why are you cutting off the ends and wasting that part of the ham?"

She says, "That's how my mom always did it." But her husband's question gets her to wondering. So she calls her mom and asks why her mom always cut the ends off the ham.

Her mom replies, "That's how my mom always did it."

So the granddaughter calls her grandma and asks, "Grandma, why did you cut off the ends of the ham?"

Her grandma answers, "We had a small oven, so I had to cut off the ends of the ham to make it fit."

Likewise, we have to consider, "Okay, that's what my parents and grandparents always did it so it must be the way it's done." Their diets and lifestyles were a certain way, and unfortunately they got stuck in an unhealthy pattern and passed it down.

Many cultures pass down their food traditions. As an example, for Italian people, pasta is part of the culture of the family. Today, gluten intolerance is a serious issue. When you eat pasta, you're making yourself unhealthy . . . possibly dangerously unhealthy.

You need to realize what's healthy for you and what isn't. You don't have to take on the diet, the lifestyle, or any of the habits of your family of origin.

Here's another story, a true one. I visited Ireland a couple years ago. Here in the United States we think, "Oh, St. Patrick's Day is when the Irish enjoy corned beef and cabbage! I'm going to do the same." But in Ireland our tour guide told me, "No, we don't eat corned beef. When our ancestors migrated to the United States during the depression, they ate corned beef, but only because they had to. Corned beef reminds us of when we were in depression days, so we don't eat it on a regular basis. You'd have to order it special at the deli, if you want it." So we in the USA wrongly link corned beef and cabbage with the Irish.

Just because history was one way, doesn't mean that way is right today.

We need to think, "Why are we doing this? Is this right? Is this healthy?" Don't base your choices on someone else's way of doing things.

We have generational oddities. I tease my mom a lot because she didn't breastfeed me. I say, "I could've been a better student and had a higher GPA if you had breastfed me, Mom!"

She answers, "I didn't know, because back then advertisements said that powdered formula was healthier than breastmilk!"

No man is ever wiser than nature or God. It's just never going to be that way. Anytime man gets a hold of it, we mess it up. Somewhere, somehow, we degrade it.

It's the same with behavior. If you grow up with a mother who's overly emotional or dramatic, you think that's normal and how you need to react to things. Or maybe you have a parent who under-reacts to matters that are serious, or reacts flippantly. Do you copy their tendencies? We can't assume that our parents' behavior or habits are ones we should emulate.

We also need to pay close attention to what our behavior and habits teach our children. Children don't analyze and weigh our behavior. They'll just become the same way because they're surrounded by it.

They unconsciously mimic their parents' behavior. Monkey see, monkey do.

I try to live the lifestyle that I want my children to live. They see me packing my lunch—that's healthier than fast food—and they see me drinking my water. They see me not drinking coffee, and not drinking things that are unhealthy.

They see me going to the gym. They see me engaging in spiritual services.

Actions speak louder than words. Our actions will always override what comes out of our mouths.

So you can't say "don't smoke" while you're smoking. You can't say "don't eat fast food" when you're eating fast food. Your actions are going to translate into their actions.

℞ Take OWNERShip—Social Health

If you want to take this step toward more vibrant health . . .

✓ To destress your family:
   ℞ Discover your children's personality types. Then you can best understand what and how they think.
   ℞ Unplug electronic devices and have "No Screen Day."
   ℞ Know your children's (and your) love languages. Read *The 5 Love Languages of Children*, *The 5 Love Languages of Teenagers*, and discover your own and your spouses in *The 5 Love Languages*, all by Gary Chapman.
✓ Live the lifestyle you want your children to live. Actions speak louder than words.

A True Test of Social Health: Boundaries

Social health also means you have to think about your boundaries—what kind of behaviors you're going to allow around you and want around you.

Unfortunately we can't pick our families. We have to identify toxic relationships that drain us. Such people just take and take. Or they make you feel bad, or down. They have a lot of negative energy.

You choose whether you take that in or not. If you allow them to make you feel bad, that's your choice.

Sometimes people shift. They can start off in a good place. Then life events happen and they become negative. Don't get me wrong—I don't say abandon them. But if you've tried to give them advice or help them and they're just dragging you down, maybe you need to limit your exposure to them. Set up boundaries. Tell them, "If you're going to talk to me and you're going to be negative, I don't want to hear it. Can we talk about something else?"

Sometimes, if you just set them straight, they will come back. Other times they won't be happy with you. Either way, you need to have those clearly set boundaries.

I have a family member who is typically angry and pessimistic. I still see this person, on occasion so they come into my space. Now, I have boundaries for my office. My office is supposed to be a healthy, healing place. When they came into my space and wanted to be gripey and negative, I had to set up boundaries. I told them, "Nope, this is a positive, healthy energy space. If you want to do that, you can go back to the car, or you can go outside, and get that out." I set this tone, "That's not accepted. It's not allowed." And it's amazing—they'll be quiet.

The same thing in my home when they come for a holiday. "Nope, we're not having that here!"

If we get repercussions and they don't want to come into our homes, we can still try to do the best we can and show them love, but we don't have to allow that kind of thing in our lives. We don't have to allow that mental abuse any more than we have to stay in a situation of physical abuse, or abuse of any kind.

You need to set that boundary. And they need to understand that there's a consequence. And if zero contact is the consequence, that's how it is.

At the same time, spend more time with the positive people in your life. Surround yourself with people who are like-minded, who have the same goals as you. They say that the people you spend most of your time with are who you become.

I've personally had this experience myself. I never wanted to be a mediocre doctor. Yes, I could just show up to my job, and I could treat people, and people would get well. But I want people not to just get well. I want them to thrive.

I could hang out with some of my colleagues who are like, "Okay, we're doing a job, and we're getting paid for what we do."

I could have decided the same. "I could go with the flow and still put my kids through college. Do I want to do that, or do I want to thrive in my career?"

I made a choice to find people who not only are doctors, but who also want to help their patients and their communities to enjoy better health. I spend time with like-minded people who want to reach even a bigger community—the United States, their country, the world. I have a big vision.

One trait I had to let go of was self-reliance. Before I found those people, I used to think I had to do this myself. That it's not good to ask for other people's help. Or I looked at others as competitors.

But when I began connecting with them, I saw that we were all working together to make things better. I finally understood that I would surely give them help if the roles were reversed.

Sometimes we just have to get out of our own way.

However, when we get advice or assistance, evaluate what they're giving you. Is this advice good, or is this bad? Is this something I'm not ready for? Does it fit my life or calling?

Also, look at those people's lifestyles. Are they living what they're talking about? If these people say they want to help people, but they're sitting in an office and not doing anything, or are letting other people do their work for them, then they're nothing but talk. If they give advice about weight loss but they're overweight, their words have no meaning.

It's hard for anybody to give advice if they're not practicing it themselves.

So look at each person's lifestyle and see if that is someone who resonates with you. If it is, then it's okay to say, "I'd like to take you out to lunch and pick your brain and make connections."

But even with positive people you may have to have boundaries. Decide for yourself how much time you're going to spend with them.

With everything in your life, learn to ask yourself, "Is this good for me" Or, "Is this good for my family?" "Is this relationship good for me? Is this relationship good for my family? Is this relationship good for my job?" "My life?"

Base your choices on thoughtful reflection, not on feelings. Feelings will often mislead you.

Social Health Success: Mentoring

You can do the same when searching for a mentor. Find a person at a higher station than you are in life, whether it be career-wise, spiritually, health-wise, or in any other way you wish to be mentored. Ask them how they got to the level they're currently at, ask about their habits, what kind of books they read, or what kind of apps they use. Call and talk with them weekly, every other week, or monthly, whatever the mentor agrees to, sometimes you have to show this person you are committed to learning and growing.

I do that a lot with my mentor. Because she's been in practice about three times longer than I have, she has a great wealth of information. Don't get me wrong—sometimes her advice resonates with me, and sometimes it doesn't. What's great is that she's fine with that! She knows I'm my own unique person.

So your mentor should identify with your uniqueness and say, "Great! I'm just subjecting this idea, and if it works, fantastic! If you tried it and it didn't work for you, give me feedback."

Social health also means find someone with less experience than you to mentor. You receive from your mentor, so give back to a mentee. Then you're receiving and also giving back.

I mentor someone who I meet with once a month. She picks my brain and asks my advice. I love it. Your mentee might actually give you a fresher perspective on things. Many times I've left the meeting and thought, "Oh wow! I went to give to her, and I got so much out of it!"

Such connections give you vitality and excitement and help you to learn and grow. Those are key benefits of good social health.

Inspire Healthy Social Change

The culture needs to change. You can start changing it, at least within your family, within your home. When you change, others are going to take notice. The sphere of your influence—your family, your friends, your community will start to change—but change starts with you. You can be the motivation for change.

Don't get me wrong—you'll get pushback. Anytime people see you making strides, they're going to try to counterbalance that, because they're not ready to make those changes. They're going to be resistant. You should rejoice in that. You should actually be thinking, "Wow, they're seeing something! So that's what's irritating them, because they're jealous." They see something that they could be doing themselves but see you doing it, and they're not ready to do it or don't want to make the effort for it.

Think of that as positive/negative feedback. You're rocking the boat, so some people around you might think, "Oh, that means if you're doing it, I could possibly do it. And I'm not ready to do it. I don't even want to do it!"

So they get a little irritated. Be bold, consistent, and committed. Because once you start changing and saying no to certain things, you're *going to* get some pushback from friends and family. They'll say, "We always did this!"

That happens a lot when stress-reducing change involves financial matters. For instance, you might step up at Christmas and say, "I'm not buying everybody a present this year because it's not financially responsible. Can we do a grab bag instead, or come up with some other way to celebrate?" You're going to get looks, at the very least.

Or you might decide, "I'm going to go gluten free." Then you go to a big family Thanksgiving dinner, and your relatives serve stuffing and a lot of other foods that you might not be able to eat. Now those people are likely to comment, "Oh, right. No stuffing. The health nut."

On the other hand, you might have friends and family who are supportive and encouraging. "She's making a life choice to improve herself. Are we going to criticize her about it, or are we going to support her?" Try to surround yourself with family, friends, and other people who will support you in your decisions and changes.

And understand that if you have to cut people loose or limit your time with those who don't support your decisions, you have to stick to your guns.

Keep inspiring healthy social change.

℞ Take OWNERShip—Social Health

If you want to take this step toward more vibrant health . . .

✓ Determine your boundaries—what kind of behaviors you're going to allow around you and want around you.
✓ If you would benefit from a relationship with a mentor, find one.
✓ If you would enjoy mentoring someone else, be one.
✓ Inspire positive change by doing good things for yourself and others.

Spiritual Health: Meditate on This and Be Uplifted

Health is physical, mental, social, and *spiritual* well-being. So we have a second S in OWNERShip: Spiritual health.

Whether or not you believe in God, research reveals that people who routinely pray or meditate tend to have better health outcomes. They tend to have better recovery times.

So cater to your spirit. Find out what it is that enables your spirit to thrive. Think about what your connection to God truly is, or what some people call Universal Intelligence—what is your connection there?

Some people connect through nature. They go for walks in the woods or in the mountains. They go out on a lake or walk along a beach near an ocean. At night, they lie in the grass and look up at the stars. That's how they connect with God or nature in their spirit and feel uplifted.

Some people feel refreshed in spirit through meditation practices. To me, meditation is simply where you're quiet and you try to tune in to your spirit, where you take time to quiet yourself and see what's going on.

That's a good test of how socially and spiritually healthy you are too. If you can't be quiet with yourself, if you need to have distractions or you need to constantly do things, then there might be something wrong. What are you trying to run away from, or hide from? What are you trying to distract yourself from?

When you take time to be quiet and refresh your spirit, you don't necessarily have to be sitting in a room or lying on a mat. Sometimes I'm just quiet in my car, with no radio on, while I'm on my way to work. I take the time to have conversations with God, and think about things, and reflect on things.

Again be mindful, be purposeful, in doing that. Pray. Meditate. It can help you be restful, positive, and can lead to moments of enlightenment.

Sometimes I feel that divine wisdom is bestowed on me when I pray, or meditate, if I take the time to listen for an answer. Many people experience the same. All of a sudden you feel like you have wisdom you didn't think you knew! I suggest you cultivate those moments.

As humans we typically want control, not to have something over us directing how we should be, or what we should do, and our spirit tends to conflict with that. Prayer and meditation are about giving up control and realizing, "Oh, there's something bigger than me and surrendering to a peaceful way of life."

Go with that stream of things. Open up to a more "whole" way of thinking. Actually, I would call it "holistic," even "universal." Not what's just good for me, but what's good for everyone, for the planet.

We talked about the light and the dark and about what feeds the light. Spiritually, the light is the Holy Spirit, God, and it helps guide everything. Feed into that Spirit. Invest in those times of prayer and meditation.

℞ Take OWNERShip—Spiritual Health

If you want to take this step toward more vibrant health . . .

✓ Find out what enables your spirit to thrive, whether it's time
   spent in nature, meditation, or prayer. Feed the light.

Healthy You, Healthy Life

Toxins accumulate in the body until they affect someone. And they
might affect different people in different ways.

I can have two patients come in with the same symptoms, and I'll
run a symptom survey on each of them, and a hair analysis on them.
They may have similar symptoms, but their hair analyses are totally
different. So I'm going to treat them totally differently, because it's a
totally different mechanism causing those symptoms.

We need to find out what their weak link is that we need to
address. One person could be sensitive to dairy. We can eliminate
dairy from their diet, and soon they're doing great! The other person
could just be magnesium deficient. "Okay, we need to increase your
magnesium." They both improve once we find out where their
weakness is in the body, where there's a stress on their system.

It's the same with chiropractic. When a patient has a misalignment
in the mid-back, the resulting pinched nerve can affect the muscle tone
of their back, their large intestines, women's ovaries, and other
functions.

Most people come in because of back pain. I can adjust the mid-
back, and the pain goes away. I also know to ask, "Have you been
having constipation issues?"

"How did you know?"

"Because that nerve that relates to your back pain also controls the large intestine as well."

Several young ladies who had pelvis misalignments were adjusted, and their cycles greatly improved. They stopped having cramps because we took the pressure off the nervous system, which let the nerves communicate effectively to the uterus and ovaries. We freed that communication up.

But that nerve could cause three distinct symptoms from the same misalignment. So everybody is different.

Perhaps surprisingly, you don't always need to pinpoint whatever is the root cause of the malfunction. You just need to eliminate the stress on the body and give it the resources to heal. Simply restore the energy with healthy choices so your body and mind can start to work better.

Our society needs restful, positive energy restored as well. Our birth vitality is almost equal to that of third-world countries, which is because doctors in the United States have changed birth into a procedure. It's no longer a natural thing of life that women naturally know how to do. Instead the medical field scares the crap out of women throughout the pregnancies. They test them, poke them, prod them, ultrasound them, worry them, and then, "Oh well, if you don't push this baby out within twelve hours, we're going to cut you open."

It's a fear experience, but culturally it's not supposed to be. It's supposed to be good, a joyous part of life.

Since a lot of my chiropractic patients are pregnant women, I encourage them, "Trust your body. You know your body. Your body is meant to do this. We are built to have babies! We are females! That's how we were born! We've been doing this for centuries."

If you are pregnant, you are built to give birth to a baby. Trust your body. Don't allow medical doctors to scare you.

Our society needs restful, positive energy restored.

It also needs ways of thinking that medical doctors aren't exposed to in medical school. We can't continue to focus on diagnosing illness, living with illness, and Band-Aiding the symptoms.

We need to focus on healing the root cause of illnesses. We need to focus on health and restoring people to vibrant health!

What we focus on, we become.

And we can't blame ill health on the genes. Identical twins have the same DNA. The same genes. One of the twins gets cancer, one does not. The one who didn't get cancer? It's because they exercised. They ate their vegetables. They focused on healthy thoughts. They were positive and energetic. They fed the health, so that negative genes don't get exposed.

The negative gene gets exposed when stress is on the body. Again, you have a choice in the environment you create for yourself, whether that environment stresses your body or helps heal you.

You have to be mindful. Step back and think, "What is healthy for me? What is healthy for my family?"

It's your health. Your future. Your life.

Take OWNERShip.

About the Author

Dr. Rachel A. Northern graduated Magna Cum Laude with a Doctor of Chiropractic degree from Palmer College of Chiropractic in Davenport, Iowa in 2003. She is certified and specializes in Activator Method, which is a specific, low force chiropractic adjustment. She is certified in Chiropractic pediatrics from ICPA. Using the Activator Method, Dr. Rachel can easily adjust all patients, from newborn babies to senior citizens, *without* twisting, turning, or "cracking" the body.

Dr. Rachel also specializes in nutrition therapy, and utilizes whole-food supplements to provide nutritional supplementation for many deficiencies in the body caused by physical, chemical, and emotional imbalances. By using symptom surveys, hair and saliva tests, she can also determine chemical toxicity, hormonal imbalances, and mineral disparities, also often treatable through nutritional supplements.

In her efforts to be actively involved in the community, she gives regular health talks and spinal screenings at various public community events. She is an active speaker on numerous health topics, such as healthy body, healthy eating, stress, detoxification/purification diets, and pediatric chiropractic.

Dr. Rachel's mission is to provide quality healthcare to all who desire it; to educate people on the body's ability to heal itself with the elimination of nervous system interference; to work in harmony with other healthcare professionals to provide the best care for the patient.

Dr. Rachel lives in Northern Illinois, with her husband and two children, and is an active member of her local community organizations and church.

Visit her online at www.TheDoctorInYou.com.

Made in the USA
Lexington, KY
25 January 2017